The Cardiovascular System at a Glance

PHILIP I. AARONSON PhD
Reader in Pharmacology
Guy's, King's and St Thomas' School of Medicine,
    Dentistry and Biomedical Sciences
King's College, London

JEREMY P.T. WARD PhD
Professor of Respiratory Cell Physiology
Guy's, King's and St Thomas' School of Medicine,
    Dentistry and Biomedical Sciences
King's College, London

CHARLES M. WIENER MD
Associate Professor of Medicine and Physiology
Johns Hopkins School of Medicine
Baltimore, MD, USA

SECOND EDITION

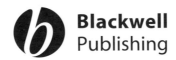

Blackwell Publishing

© 1999, 2004 by Blackwell Publishing Ltd

Blackwell Publishing, Inc., 350 Main Street, Malden, Massachusetts 02148-5020, USA
Blackwell Publishing Ltd, 9600 Garsington Road, Oxford OX4 2DQ, UK
Blackwell Publishing Asia Pty Ltd, 550 Swanston Street, Carlton, Victoria 3053, Australia

First published 1999
Reprinted 2000, 2001
Second edition 2004

Library of Congress Cataloging-in-Publication Data
Aaronson, Philip Irving, 1953–
    The cardiovascular system at a glance / Philip I. Aaronson, Jeremy P.T. Ward, Charles M.
Wiener.— 2nd ed.
        p. ; cm.
Previous ed. published in 1999, entered under title.
Includes index.
    ISBN 1-4051-1327-8
    1. Cardiovascular system—Physiology.   2. Cardiovascular system—Pathophysiology.
    [DNLM: 1. Cardiovascular System—anatomy & histology.   2. Cardiovascular Diseases.   3.
Cardiovascular Physiology.   WG 100 A113c 2004]   I. Ward, Jeremy P.T.   II. Wiener, Charles M.
III. Cardiovascular system at a glance.   IV. Title.
    QP101.C293 2004
    616.1—dc21

                                                                        2003012546

A catalogue record for this title is available from the British Library

Set in 9/11.5 Times by Graphicraft Limited, Hong Kong
Printed and bound by Replika Press Pvt. Ltd, India

Commissioning Editor: Fiona Goodgame
Managing Editor: Geraldine Jeffers
Editorial Assistant: Nicola Ulyatt
Production Editor: Fiona Pattison
Production Controller: Kate Charman

For further information on Blackwell Publishing, visit our website:
http://www.blackwellpublishing.com

Contents

Preface

This book aims to provide a comprehensive yet concise revision aid to the cardiovascular system, integrating normal structure, function and regulation with pathophysiology, pharmacology and therapeutics. It is primarily aimed towards medical students in their early years, and should be particularly useful to those taking systems- or case-based courses where the basic science is interwoven with clinical examples. The incorporation of basic clinical material covering key cardiovascular diseases should also make this book useful to students of nursing and other healthcare professions.

As with other volumes in the At a Glance series, the book is based around two page spreads for each topic, loosely equivalent to the amount of material normally presented in a lecture. Case studies based on important and commonly encountered conditions are also provided, and are selected so that they can be used both basic science and clinical study. Although primarily designed for revision and an adjunct to course materials, the book covers all the core elements of the cardiovascular system and its major diseases, and as such could be used as a main text in the early years of the course. It is advised, however, that reference to more detailed textbooks will aid deeper and wider understanding of the subject. This is particularly the case for the clinical sections of the book, which are necessarily limited in a volume of this size.

In this second edition we have updated the text and in some cases extended the content, for example the new chapter on anti-coagulatants and thrombolytics, whereas elsewhere the content has been refined and simplified to make understanding easier. We have also corrected several errors that previously escaped our notice in the first edition. We would like to thank our colleagues for helpful and invaluable advice during the production of this edition, particularly Dr Jane Ward, and the many students who have advised us on how to make the book easier to understand, and have pointed out errors. We would also like to thank all the staff at Blackwell Publishing for their support and encouragement, particularly the long suffering and very wonderful Geraldine Jeffers, and our production editor Fiona Pattison who put it all together.

Recommended reading

J.R. Levick. An Introduction to Cardiovascular Physiology. 4th edition. Arnold, London, 2003.

E. Braunwald, D. Ziper, P. Libby, eds. Heart Disease: A textbook of Cardiovascular Medicine. 6th Edition. WB Saunders, Philadelphia, 2001.

Sources of illustrations

Fig. 2.1(d) Reproduced from *J Cell Biol*, 1969; **42**: 1–45 by copyright permission of The Rockefeller University Press.

Fig. 3.1 (top) Reproduced with permission from Gosling JA *et al. Human Anatomy—color atlas and text*, 3rd edn. Mosby Wolfe, London, 1996.

Fig. 4.1(a) Reproduced with permission from Berne RM. *Handbook of Physiology.* Oxford University Press, New York, 1980.

Fig. 17.2 Reproduced with permission from Berne RM & Levy MN. *Cardiovascular Physiology*, 2nd edn. Mosby, St Louis, 1972.

Fig. 18.1 (inset) Reproduced with permission from McDonald DA. *Blood Flow in Arteries*, 2nd edn. Edward Arnold, London, 1974.

Fig. 29.1(a) Reproduced with permission from Berne RM, Levy MN. *Cardiovascular Physiology*, 5th edn. Mosby, St Louis, 1986.

Table 29.1 Reproduced with permission from Mitchell JH, Blomqvist G. Maximal oxygen uptake. *N Engl J Med* 1971; **284**: 1018. © Massachusetts Medical Society. All rights reserved.

Fig. 38.1 (top right) Reproduced with permission from Chiodo CP, Carlson W, Lilly LS. Ischaemic heart disease. Lilly LS, ed. *Pathophysiology of Heart Disease*. Lea & Febiger, Philadelphia, 1993.

Fig. 39.1 Reproduced in part with permission from Opie LH, ed. *Drugs for the Heart*, 3rd edn. WB Saunders, Philadelphia, 1991.

1 Overview of the cardiovascular system

The following labels appear on the figure:

- Blood loses CO_2, gains oxygen
- Pulmonary circulation
- Right atrium
- Vena caval pressure = 0
- Less oxygenated blood
  - ~70% saturated
- **Veins**
  - thin walled
  - distensible
  - contain 70% of blood
  - blood reservoirs
  - return blood to the heart
- Portal vein
- Venous valves (prevent backflux of blood)
- Renal circulation
- Venules and veins collect blood from exchange vessels
- Head and neck arteries
- Arm arteries
- Bronchial arteries
- Right ventricle
- Coronary circulation
- Trunk arteries
- Hepatic artery
- Liver
- Efferent arterioles
- Afferent arterioles
- Splenic artery
- Mesenteric arteries
- Left atrium
- Left ventricle
- **Aortic pressure**
  - systolic = 120
  - diastolic = 80
  - mean = 93
- **Elastic artery**
  - recoil helps propel blood during diastole
- **Arterial system**
  - contains 17% of blood
  - distributes blood throughout the body
  - dampens pulsations in blood pressure and flow
- **Highly oxygenated blood**
  - ~98% saturated
- Pelvic and leg arteries
- Resistance arteries regulate flow of blood to the exchange vessels
- **Capillaries and postcapillary venules**
  - exchange vessels
  - blood loses O_2 to tissues
  - tissues lose CO_2 and waste products to blood
  - immune cells can enter tissues via postcapillary venules

1.1

The cardiovascular system is composed of the heart, blood vessels and blood. In simple terms, its main functions are:

1 Distribution of O_2 and nutrients (e.g. glucose, amino acids) to all body tissues.

2 Transportation of CO_2 and metabolic waste products (e.g. urea) from the tissues to the lungs and excretory organs.

3 Distribution of water, electrolytes and hormones throughout the body.

4 Contributing to the infrastructure of the immune system.

5 Thermoregulation.

Blood is composed of **plasma**, an aqueous solution containing electrolytes, proteins and other molecules, in which **cells** are suspended. The cells comprise 40–45% of blood volume and are mainly **erythrocytes**, but also **white blood cells**

and **platelets**. Blood volume is about 5.5 L in an 'average' 70-kg man.

Figure 1.1 illustrates the 'plumbing' of the cardiovascular system.

Blood is driven through the cardiovascular system by the **heart**, a muscular pump divided into left and right sides. Each side contains two chambers, an **atrium** and a **ventricle**, composed mainly of cardiac muscle cells. The thin-walled atria serve to fill or 'prime' the thick-walled ventricles, which when full constrict forcefully, creating a pressure head that drives the blood out into the body. Blood enters and leaves each chamber of the heart through separate one-way valves, which open and close reciprocally (i.e. one closes before the other opens) to ensure that flow is unidirectional.

Consider the flow of blood, starting with its exit from the left ventricle.

When the ventricles contract, the left ventricular internal pressure rises from 0 to 120 mmHg (atmospheric pressure = 0). As the pressure rises, the aortic valve opens and blood is expelled into the **aorta**, the first and largest artery of the **systemic circulation**. This period of ventricular contraction is termed **systole**. The maximal pressure during systole is called the **systolic pressure**, and it serves both to drive blood through the aorta and to distend the aorta, which is quite elastic. The aortic valve then closes, and the left ventricle relaxes so that it can be refilled with blood from the left atrium via the mitral valve. The period of relaxation is called **diastole**. During diastole aortic blood flow and pressure diminish but do not fall to zero, because *elastic recoil* of the aorta continues to exert a **diastolic pressure** on the blood, which gradually falls to a minimum level of about 80 mmHg. The difference between systolic and diastolic pressures is termed the **pulse pressure**. **Mean aortic pressure** is pressure averaged over the entire cardiac cycle. Because the heart spends approximately 60% of the cardiac cycle in diastole, the mean aortic pressure is approximately equal to the diastolic pressure + one-third of the pulse pressure, rather than to the arithmetic average of the systolic and diastolic pressures.

The blood flows from the aorta into the **major arteries**, each of which supplies blood to an organ or body region. These arteries divide and subdivide into smaller **muscular arteries**, which eventually give rise to the **arterioles**—arteries with diameters of < 100 μm. Blood enters the arterioles at a mean pressure of about 60–70 mmHg.

The walls of the arteries and arterioles have circumferentially arranged layers of **smooth muscle cells**. The lumen of the entire vascular system is lined by a monolayer of **endothelial cells**. These cells secrete vasoactive substances and serve as a barrier, restricting and controlling the movement of fluid, molecules and cells into and out of the vasculature.

The arterioles lead to the smallest vessels, the **capillaries**, which form a dense network within all body tissues. The capillary wall is a layer of overlapping endothelial cells, with no smooth muscle cells. The pressure in the capillaries ranges from about 25 mmHg on the arterial side to 15 mmHg at the venous end. The capillaries converge into small **venules**, which also have thin walls of mainly endothelial cells. The venules merge into larger venules, with an increasing content of smooth muscle cells as they widen. These then converge to become **veins**, which progressively join to give rise to the **superior** and **inferior venae cavae**, through which blood returns to the right side of the heart. Veins have a larger diameter than arteries, and thus offer relatively little resistance to flow. The small pressure gradient between venules (15 mmHg) and the venae cavae (0 mmHg) is therefore sufficient to drive blood back to the heart.

Blood from the venae cavae enters the **right atrium**, and then the **right ventricle** through the **tricuspid valve**. Contraction of the right ventricle, simultaneous with that of the left ventricle, forces blood through the pulmonary valve into the pulmonary artery, which progressively subdivides to form the arteries, arterioles and capillaries of the **pulmonary circulation**. The pulmonary circulation is shorter and has a much lower pressure than the systemic circulation, with systolic and diastolic pressures of about 25 and 10 mmHg, respectively. The pulmonary capillary network within the lungs surrounds the alveoli of the lungs, allowing exchange of CO_2 for O_2. Oxygenated blood enters pulmonary venules and veins, and then the **left atrium**, which pumps it into the left ventricle for the next systemic cycle.

The output of the right ventricle is slightly lower than that of the left ventricle. This is because 1–2% of the systemic blood flow never reaches the right atrium, but is shunted to the left side of the heart via the bronchial circulation (Fig. 1.1) and a small fraction of coronary blood flow drains into the thebesian veins (see Chapter 24).

Blood vessel functions

Each vessel type has important functions in addition to being a conduit for blood.

The branching system of elastic and muscular arteries progressively reduces the pulsations in blood pressure and flow imposed by the intermittent ventricular contractions.

The smallest arteries and arterioles play a crucial role in regulating the amount of blood flowing to the tissues by dilating or constricting. This function is regulated by the sympathetic nervous system, and factors generated locally in tissues. These vessels are referred to as **resistance arteries**, because their constriction resists the flow of blood.

Capillaries and small venules are the **exchange vessels**. Through their walls, gases, fluids and molecules are transferred between blood and tissues. White blood cells can also pass through the venule walls to fight infection in the tissues.

Venules can constrict to offer resistance to the bloodflow, and the ratio of arteriolar and venular resistance exerts an important influence on the movement of fluid between capillaries and tissues, thereby affecting blood volume.

The veins are thin walled and very *distensible*, and therefore contain about 70% of all blood in the cardiovascular system. The arteries contain just 17% of total blood volume. Veins and venules thus serve as volume reservoirs, which can shift blood from the peripheral circulation into the heart and arteries by constricting. In doing so, they are able to increase the **cardiac output** (volume of blood pumped by the heart per unit time), and they are also able to maintain the blood pressure and tissue perfusion in essential organs if **haemorrhage** (blood loss) occurs.

2 Gross anatomy and histology of the heart

2.1

Gross anatomy of the heart (Fig. 2.1a)

The heart consists of four chambers. Blood flows into the right atrium via the superior and inferior venae cavae. The left and right atria connect to the ventricles via the mitral (two cusps) and tricuspid (three cusps) atrioventricular (AV) valves, respectively. The AV valves are passive and close when the ventricular pressure exceeds that in the atrium. They are prevented from being everted into the atria during systole by fine cords (**chordae tendineae**) attached between the free margins of the cusps and the papillary muscles, which contract during systole. The outflow from the right ventricle passes through the pulmonary semilunar valve to the pulmonary artery, and that from the left ventricle enters the aorta via the aortic semilunar valve. These valves close passively at the end of systole, when ventricular pressure falls below that of the arteries. Both semilunar valves have three cusps.

The cusps or leaflets of the cardiac valves are formed of fibrous connective tissue, covered in a thin layer of cells similar to and contiguous with the **endocardium** (AV valves and ventricular surface of semilunar valves) and **endothelium** (vascular side of semilunar valves). When closed, the cusps form a tight seal (come to apposition) at the **commissures** (line at which the edges of the leaflets meet).

The atria and ventricles are separated by a band of fibrous connective tissue called the **annulus fibrosus**, which provides a skeleton for attachment of the muscle and insertion of the valves. It also prevents electrical conduction between the atria and ventricles except at the **atrioventricular node** (AVN). This is situated near the interatrial septum and the mouth of the coronary sinus and is an important element of the cardiac electrical conduction system.

The ventricles fill during diastole; at the initiation of the heart beat the atria contract and complete ventricular filling. As the ventricles contract the pressure rises sharply, closing the AV valves. When ventricular pressure exceeds the pulmonary artery or aortic pressure, the semilunar valves open and ejection occurs (see Chapter 13). As systole ends and ventricular pressure falls, the semilunar valves are closed by backflow of blood from the arteries.

The force of contraction is generated by the muscle of the heart, the **myocardium**. The atrial walls are thin. The greater pressure generated by the left ventricle compared with the right is reflected by its greater wall thickness. The inside of the heart is covered in a thin layer of cells called the **endocardium**, which is similar to the endothelium of blood vessels. The outer surface of the myocardium is covered by the **epicardium**, a layer of mesothelial cells. The whole heart is enclosed in the **pericardium**, a thin fibrous sheath or sac, which prevents excessive enlargement. The **pericardial space** contains interstitial fluid as a lubricant.

Structure of the myocardium

The myocardium consists of **cardiac myocytes** (*muscle cells*) that show a striated subcellular structure, although they are less organized than skeletal muscle. The cells are relatively small ($100 \times 20\ \mu m$) and branched, with a single nucleus, and are rich in mitochondria. They are connected together as a network by **intercalated discs** (Fig. 2.1b), where the cell membranes are closely opposed. The intercalated discs provide both a structural attachment by 'glueing' the cells together at **desmosomes**, and an electrical connection through **gap junctions** formed of pores made up of proteins called **connexons**. As a result, the myocardium acts as a **functional syncytium**, in other words as a single functional unit, even though the individual cells are still separate. The gap junctions play a vital role in conduction of the electrical impulse through the myocardium (see Chapter 15).

The myocytes contain **actin** and **myosin** filaments which form the contractile apparatus, and exhibit the classical M and Z lines and A, H and I bands (Fig. 2.1c). The intercalated discs always coincide with a Z line, as it is here that the actin filaments are anchored to the cytoskeleton. At the Z lines the **sarcolemma** (cell membrane) forms tubular invaginations into the cells known as the **transverse (T) tubular system**. The **sarcoplasmic reticulum** (SR) is less extensive than in skeletal muscle, and runs generally in parallel with the length of the cell (Fig. 2.1d). Close to the T tubules the SR forms **terminal cisternae** that with the T tubule make up **diads** (Fig. 2.1e), an important component of excitation–contraction coupling (see Chapter 11). The typical *triad* seen in skeletal muscle is less often present. The T tubules and SR never physically join, but are separated by a narrow gap. The myocardium has an extensive system of capillaries.

Coronary circulation (Fig. 2.1f)

The heart has a rich blood supply, derived from the **left and right coronary arteries**. These arise separately from the aortic sinus at the base of the aorta, behind the cusps of the aortic valve. They are not blocked by the cusps during systole because of eddy currents, and remain patent throughout the cardiac cycle. The **right coronary artery** runs forward between the pulmonary trunk and right atrium, to the AV sulcus. As it descends to the lower margin of the heart, it divides to **posterior descending** and **right marginal** branches. The **left coronary artery** runs behind the pulmonary trunk and forward between it and the left atrium. It divides into the **circumflex**, **left marginal** and **anterior descending** branches. There are anastomoses between the left and right marginal branches, and the anterior and posterior descending arteries, although these are not sufficient to maintain perfusion if one side of the coronary circulation is occluded.

Most of the blood returns to the right atrium via the **coronary sinus**, and **anterior cardiac veins**. The **large** and **small** coronary veins run parallel to the left and right coronary arteries, respectively, and empty into the sinus. Numerous other small vessels empty into the cardiac chambers directly, including **thebesian veins** and **arteriosinusoidal vessels**.

The coronary circulation is capable of developing a good collateral system in ischaemic heart disease, when a branch or branches are occluded by, for example, atheromatous plaques. Most of the left ventricle is supplied by the left coronary artery, and occlusion can therefore be very dangerous. The AVN and **sinus node** are supplied by the right coronary artery in the majority of people; disease in this artery can cause a slow heart rate and AV block (see Chapters 10, 15).

3 Vascular anatomy

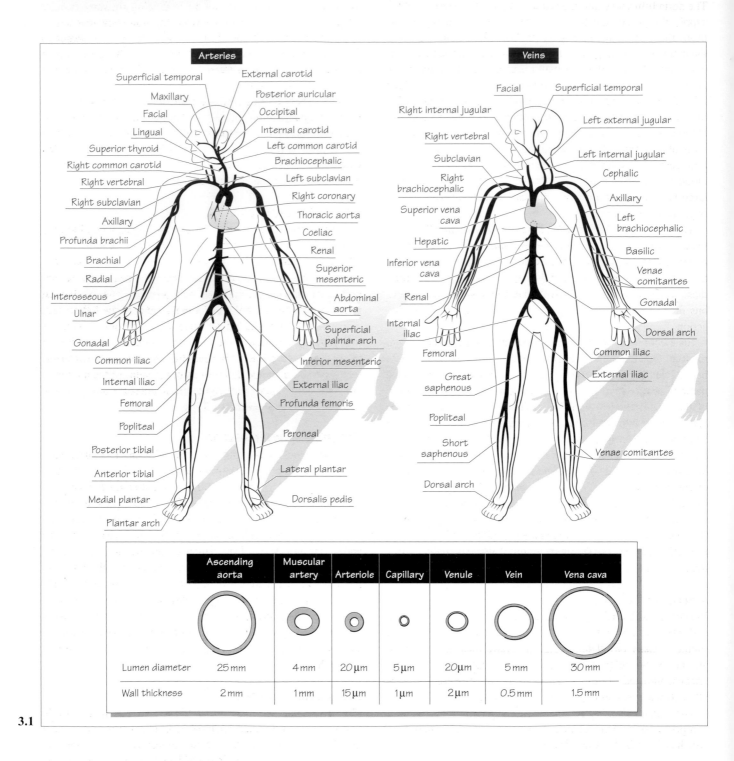

	Ascending aorta	Muscular artery	Arteriole	Capillary	Venule	Vein	Vena cava
Lumen diameter	25 mm	4 mm	20 μm	5 μm	20μm	5 mm	30 mm
Wall thickness	2 mm	1 mm	15 μm	1μm	2μm	0.5 mm	1.5 mm

3.1

The blood vessels of the cardiovascular system are for conveni-ence of description classified into **arteries** (elastic and muscular), **resistance vessels** (small arteries and arterioles), **capillaries**, **venules** and **veins**. Typical dimensions for the different types of vessel are illustrated.

The systemic circulation
Arteries
The **systemic (or greater) circulation** begins with the pumping of blood by the left ventricle into the largest artery, the **aorta**. This ascends from the top of the heart, bends downward at

the *aortic arch* and descends just anterior to the spinal column. The aorta bifurcates into the left and right *iliac arteries*, which supply the pelvis and legs. The major arteries supplying the head, the arms and the heart arise from the aortic arch, and the main arteries supplying the visceral organs branch from the descending aorta. All of the major organs except the liver (see below) are therefore supplied with blood by arteries which arise from the aorta. The fundamentally *parallel* organization of the systemic vasculature has a number of advantages over the alternative *series* arrangement, in which blood would flow sequentially through one organ after another. The parallel arrangement of the vascular system ensures that the supply of blood to each organ is relatively independent, is driven by a large pressure head, and also that each organ receives highly oxygenated blood.

The aorta and its major branches (**brachiocephalic, common carotid, subclavian** and **common iliac** arteries) are termed **elastic arteries**. In addition to conducting blood away from the heart, these arteries distend during systole and recoil during diastole, damping the pulse wave and evening out the discontinuous flow of blood created by the heart's intermittent pumping action.

Elastic arteries branch to give rise to **muscular arteries** with relatively thicker walls; this prevents their collapse when joints bend. The muscular arteries give rise to **resistance vessels**, so named because they present the greatest part of the resistance of the vasculature to the flow of blood. These are sometimes subclassified into *small arteries*, which have multiple layers of smooth muscle cells in their walls, and **arterioles**, which have one or two layers of smooth muscle cells. Resistance vessels have the highest wall/lumen ratio in the vasculature. The degree of constriction or **tone** of these vessels regulates the amount of blood flowing to each small area of tissue. All but the smallest resistance vessels tend to be heavily innervated (especially in the *splanchnic, renal* and *cutaneous* vasculatures) by the **sympathetic nervous system**, the activity of which usually causes them to constrict (see Chapter 27).

Arterial anastomoses

In addition to branching to give rise to smaller vessels, arteries and arterioles may also merge to form **anastomoses**. These are found in many circulations (e.g. the brain, mesentery, uterus, around joints) and provide an alternative supply of blood if one artery is blocked. If this occurs, the anastamosing artery gradually enlarges, providing a **collateral circulation**.

The smallest arterioles, capillaries and postcapillary venules comprise the **microcirculation**, the structure and function of which is described in Chapters 19 and 20.

Veins

The venous system can be divided into the **venules**, which contain one or two layers of smooth muscle cells, and the **veins**. The veins of the limbs, particularly the legs, contain paired semilunar **valves** which ensure that the blood cannot move backwards. These are orientated so that they are pressed against the venous wall when the blood is flowing forward, but are forced out to occlude the lumen when the blood flow reverses.

The veins from the head, neck and arms come together to form the **superior vena cava**, and those from the lower part of the body merge into the **inferior vena cava**. These deliver blood to the right atrium, which pumps it into the right ventricle.

The one or two veins draining a body region typically run next to the artery supplying that region. This promotes heat conservation, because at low temperatures the warmer arterial blood gives up its heat to the cooler venous blood, rather than to the external environment. The pulsations of the artery caused by the heart beat also aid the venous flow of blood.

The pulmonary circulation

The **pulmonary (or lesser) circulation** begins when blood is pumped by the right ventricle into the *main pulmonary artery*, which immediately bifurcates into the *right* and *left pulmonary arteries* supplying each lung. This 'venous' blood is oxygenated during its passage through the pulmonary capillaries. It then returns to the heart via the *pulmonary veins* to the left atrium, which pumps it into the left ventricle. The metabolic demands of the lungs are not met by the pulmonary circulation, but by the **bronchial circulation**. This arises from the *intercostal arteries*, which branch from the aorta. Most of the veins of the bronchial circulation terminate in the right atrium, but some drain into the pulmonary veins (see Chapter 25).

The splanchnic circulation

The arrangement of the **splanchnic circulation** (liver and digestive organs) is a partial exception to the parallel organization of the systemic vasculature (see Fig. 1.1). Although a fraction of the blood supply to the liver is provided by the hepatic artery, the liver receives most (~70%) of its blood via the *portal vein*. This vessel carries venous blood that has passed through the capillary beds of the stomach, spleen, pancreas and intestine. Most of the liver's circulation is therefore *in series* with that of the digestive organs. This arrangement facilitates hepatic uptake of nutrients and detoxification of foreign substances which have been absorbed during digestion. This type of sequential perfusion of two capillary beds is referred to as a **portal circulation**. A somewhat different type of portal circulation is also found within the kidney.

The lymphatic system

The body contains a parallel circulatory system of **lymphatic vessels** and **nodes** (see Chapter 19). The lymphatic system functions to return to the cardiovascular system the approximately 8 L/day of interstitial fluid that leaves the exchange vessels to enter body tissues. The larger lymphatic vessels pass through nodes containing lymphocytes, which act to mount an immune response to microbes, bacterial toxins and other foreign material carried into the lymphatic system with the interstitial fluid.

4 Vascular histology and smooth muscle cell ultrastructure

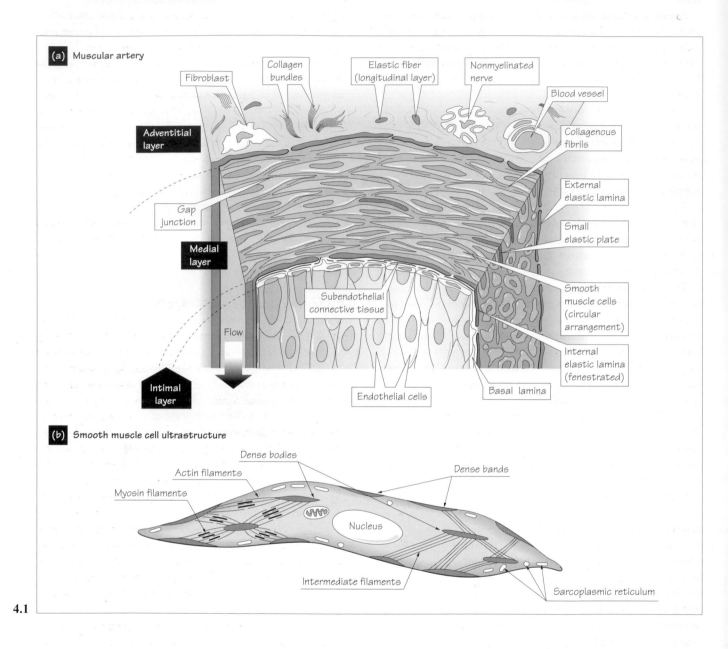

(a) Muscular artery

- Fibroblast
- Collagen bundles
- Elastic fiber (longitudinal layer)
- Nonmyelinated nerve
- Blood vessel
- Collagenous fibrils
- External elastic lamina
- Small elastic plate
- Smooth muscle cells (circular arrangement)
- Internal elastic lamina (fenestrated)
- Basal lamina
- Endothelial cells
- Subendothelial connective tissue
- Gap junction
- Flow

Adventitial layer

Medial layer

Intimal layer

(b) Smooth muscle cell ultrastructure

- Dense bodies
- Dense bands
- Actin filaments
- Myosin filaments
- Nucleus
- Intermediate filaments
- Sarcoplasmic reticulum

4.1

Larger blood vessels share a common three-layered structure. Figure 4.1(a) illustrates the arrangement of these layers, or *tunics*, in a muscular artery.

A thin inner layer, the **tunica intima**, comprises an *endothelial cell* monolayer (*endothelium*) supported by connective tissue. The endothelial cells lining the vascular lumen are sealed to each other by *tight junctions*, which restrict the diffusion of large molecules across the endothelium. The endothelial cells play a crucial role in controlling vascular permeability, vasoconstriction, angiogenesis (growth of new blood vessels) and regulation of haemostasis. The intima is relatively thicker in larger arteries, and contains some smooth muscle cells in large and medium-sized arteries and veins.

The thick middle layer, the **tunica media**, is separated from the intima by a fenestrated (perforated) sheath, the *internal elastic lamina*, mostly composed of elastin. The media contains *smooth muscle cells* embedded in an extracellular matrix composed mainly of collagen, elastin and proteoglycans. The cells are shaped like elongated and irregular spindles or cylinders with tapering ends, and are 15–100 μm long. In the arterial system, they are orientated circularly or in a low-pitch spiral, so that the vascular lumen is narrowed when they contract. Individual cells are long enough to wrap around small arterioles several times.

Adjacent smooth muscle cells form **gap junctions**. These are areas of close cellular contact in which arrays of large channels called **connexons** span both cell membranes, allowing ions to flow from one cell to the other. The smooth muscle cells therefore form a **syncitium**, in which depolarization spreads from each cell to its neighbours.

An *external elastic lamina* separates the tunica media from the outer layer, the **tunica adventitia**. This contains collagenous tissue supporting *fibroblasts* and *nerves*. In large arteries and veins, the adventitia contains **vasa vasorum**, small blood vessels which also penetrate into the outer portion of the media and supply the vascular wall with oxygen and nutrients.

Although arteries and veins share the basic three-layered structure, the layers are less distinct in the venous system. Compared to arteries, veins have a thinner tunica media containing a smaller amount of smooth muscle cells, which also tend to have a more random orientation.

The protein **elastin** is found mainly in the arteries. Molecules of elastin are arranged into a network of randomly coiled fibres. These molecular 'springs' allow arteries to expand during systole and then rebound during diastole to keep the blood flowing forward. This is particularly important in the aorta and other large elastic arteries, in which the media contains fenestrated sheets of elastin separating the smooth muscle cells into multiple concentric layers (**lamellae**).

The fibrous protein **collagen** is present in all three layers of the vascular wall, and functions as a framework that anchors the smooth muscle cells in place. At high internal pressures, the collagen network becomes very rigid, limiting vascular distensibility. This is particularly important in veins, which have a higher collagen content than arteries.

Exchange vessel structure

Capillaries and postcapillary venules are tubes formed of a single layer of overlapping endothelial cells. This is supported and surrounded on the external side by the *basal lamina*, a 50–100 nm-thick layer of fibrous proteins including collagen, and glycoproteins. *Pericytes*, isolated cells which can give rise to smooth muscle cells during angiogenesis, adhere to the outside of the basal lamina, especially in postcapillary venules. The luminal side of the endothelium is coated by *glycocalyx*, a dense glycoprotein network attached to the cell membrane.

There are three types of capillaries, and these differ in their locations and permeabilities. Their structures are illustrated in Chapter 19.

Continuous capillaries occur in skin, muscles, lungs and the central nervous system. They have a low permeability to molecules that cannot pass readily through cell membranes, owing to the presence of tight junctions which bring the overlapping membranes of adjacent endothelial cells into close contact. The

tight junctions run around the perimeter of each cell, forming a seal restricting the paracellular flow of molecules of molecular weight (MW) > 10 000. These junctions are especially tight in most capillaries of the central nervous system, and form an integral part of the **blood–brain barrier** (see Chapter 19).

Fenestrated capillaries are much more permeable than continuous capillaries. These are found in endocrine glands, renal glomeruli, intestinal villi and other tissues in which large amounts of fluid or metabolites enter or leave capillaries. In addition to having leakier intercellular junctions, the endothelial cells of these capillaries contain *fenestrae*, circular pores of diameter 50–100 nm spanning areas of the cells where the cytoplasm is thinned. Except in the renal glomeruli, fenestrae are usually covered by a thin perforated diaphragm.

Discontinuous capillaries or **sinusoids** are found in liver, spleen and bone marrow. These are large irregularly shaped capillaries with gaps between the endothelial cells wide enough to allow large proteins and even erythrocytes to cross the capillary wall.

Smooth muscle cell ultrastructure

The cytoplasm of vascular smooth muscle cells contains thin **actin** and thick **myosin** filaments (Fig. 4.1b). Instead of being aligned into sarcomeres as in cardiac myocytes, groups of actin filaments running roughly parallel to the long axis of the cell are anchored at one end into elongated **dense bodies** in the cytoplasm and **dense bands** along the inner face of the cell membrane. Dense bodies and bands are linked by bundles of **intermediate filaments** composed mainly of the proteins **desmin** and **vimentin** to form the **cytoskeleton**, an internal scaffold giving the cell its shape. The free ends of the actin filaments interdigitate with myosin filaments. The myosin crossbridges are structured so that the actin filaments on either side of a myosin filament are pulled in opposite directions during crossbridge cycling. This draws the dense bodies towards each other, causing the cytoskeleton, and therefore the cell, to become shorter and fatter. The dense bands are attached to the extracellular matrix by membrane-spanning **integrins**, allowing force development to be distributed through the entire vascular wall.

The **sarcoplasmic reticulum** (SR, also termed smooth endoplasmic reticulum) occupies 2–6% of cell volume. This network of tubes and flattened sacs permeates the cell and contains a high concentration (~50 mmol/L) of Ca^{2+}. Elements of the SR closely approach the cell membrane. Several types of Ca^{2+}-regulated ion channels and transporters have been found to be concentrated in these areas of the plasmalemma, which may have an important role in cellular excitation.

The nucleus is located in the central part of the cell. Organelles including rough endoplasmic reticulum, Golgi complex and mitochondria are mainly found in the perinuclear region.

5 Constituents of blood

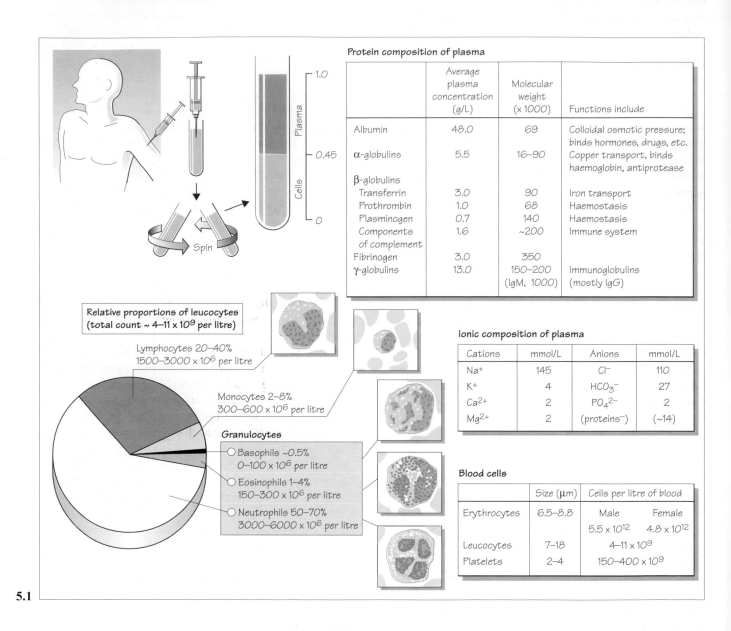

Protein composition of plasma

	Average plasma concentration (g/L)	Molecular weight (x 1000)	Functions include
Albumin	48.0	69	Colloidal osmotic pressure; binds hormones, drugs, etc.
α-globulins	5.5	16–90	Copper transport, binds haemoglobin, antiprotease
β-globulins			
Transferrin	3.0	90	Iron transport
Prothrombin	1.0	68	Haemostasis
Plasminogen	0.7	140	Haemostasis
Components of complement	1.6	~200	Immune system
Fibrinogen	3.0	350	
γ-globulins	13.0	150–200 (IgM, 1000)	Immunoglobulins (mostly IgG)

Relative proportions of leucocytes (total count ~ 4–11 x 10⁹ per litre)

Lymphocytes 20–40%
1500–3000 x 10⁶ per litre

Monocytes 2–8%
300–600 x 10⁶ per litre

Granulocytes
- Basophils ~0.5%
  0–100 x 10⁶ per litre
- Eosinophils 1–4%
  150–300 x 10⁶ per litre
- Neutrophils 50–70%
  3000–6000 x 10⁶ per litre

Ionic composition of plasma

Cations	mmol/L	Anions	mmol/L
Na⁺	145	Cl⁻	110
K⁺	4	HCO₃⁻	27
Ca²⁺	2	PO₄²⁻	2
Mg²⁺	2	(proteins⁻)	(~14)

Blood cells

	Size (μm)	Cells per litre of blood	
		Male	Female
Erythrocytes	6.5–8.8	5.5 x 10¹²	4.8 x 10¹²
Leucocytes	7–18	4–11 x 10⁹	
Platelets	2–4	150–400 x 10⁹	

5.1

The primary function of blood is to deliver O_2 and energy sources to the tissues, and to remove CO_2 and waste products. It contains important elements of the defence and immune systems, is important for the regulation of temperature, and transports hormones and other signalling molecules between tissues. In a 70-kg man blood volume is ~5500 ml, or 8% of body weight. Blood consists of **plasma** and **blood cells**. If 100 ml of blood is spun in a centrifuge, the cells sediment and this **packed cell volume** (PCV, haematocrit) is normally ~45 ml (0.45) in men, less (~0.42) in women.

Plasma

The plasma volume is ~5% of the body weight. It consists of ions in solution and a wide range of plasma proteins. After clotting a straw-coloured fluid called **serum** remains, which differs from plasma only in that fibrinogen and other clotting factors have been removed. The plasma has an **osmolarity** of ~300 mosmol/L, mostly due to the dissolved ions and small diffusible molecules (glucose and urea). These diffusible entities exert the **crystalloid osmotic pressure**. Proteins do not pass through capillary walls easily, and are responsible for the **colloidal osmotic pressure** (or **oncotic** pressure) of the plasma. This has a normal value of ~25 mmHg, and is critical for fluid transfer across the capillary wall. Maintenance of plasma osmolarity is vital for the regulation of tissue cell volume and blood volume. Increased crystalloid osmotic pressure stimulates reabsorption of water by the kidney, and increases in blood volume. Decreased colloidal osmotic pressure (e.g. low plasma albumin) reduces reabsorption of fluid from tissues back into the blood, and leads to **oedema** (see Chapter 20).

Ionic composition

Na^+ is the most prevalent ion in the plasma, and the main determinant of plasma osmolarity and thus blood volume. The concentration of the major ions is shown in Fig. 5.1, but others are present in smaller amounts (e.g. trace elements). Changes in ionic concentration can have major consequences for excitable tissues (e.g. K^+, Ca^{2+}). Na^+, K^+ and Cl^- are completely dissociated in the plasma, but Ca^{2+} and Mg^{2+} are partly bound to plasma proteins, so that free concentration is ~50% of the total.

Proteins

Normal total plasma protein concentration is 65–83 g/L; as proteins vary widely in molecular weight the molar concentration is an approximation. Most plasma proteins other than γ-globulins (see below) are synthesized in the liver. Proteins can ionize as either acids or bases because of the presence of both NH_2 and COOH groups. At pH 7.4 they are mostly in the anionic (acidic) form. Their ability to accept or donate H^+ means they can act as buffers, although they account for only ~15% of the buffering capacity of blood. Plasma proteins have an important transport function. They bind with many hormones (e.g. cortisol and thyroxine) and metals (e.g. iron), and are important for blood transport of many drugs, to which they also bind. They may therefore modulate the free concentration of such agents, and thus their biological activity.

Types of plasma protein

Plasma proteins are classified into **albumin** (~48 g/L), **globulin** (~25 g/L) and **fibrinogen** (~2–4 g/L) fractions. Globulins are further classified as α-, β- and γ-globulins, each of which may include many different proteins. β-globulins include transferrin (iron transport), components of complement (immune system), and prothrombin and plasminogen, which with fibrinogen are involved in blood clotting (see Chapter 7). The most important γ-globulins are the immunoglobulins.

Blood cells

In the adult, all blood cells are produced in the **red bone marrow**, although in the fetus, and following bone marrow damage in the adult, they are also produced in the liver and spleen. The marrow contains a small number of **uncommitted stem cells**, which differentiate into specific **committed stem cells** for each blood cell type. The average number of the main types of cell is shown in the Fig. 5.1.

Erythrocytes

Erythrocytes (red cells) are by far the most numerous cells in the blood, with ~5.5×10^{12}/L in males (red cell count, RCC).

The haemoglobin they contain is responsible for carriage of O_2, and plays an important role in acid–base buffering. Erythrocytes are biconcave discs and have no nucleus. Their shape and flexibility allows them to deform easily and pass through the capillaries. The **erythrocyte sedimentation rate (ESR)** is the rate at which cells sediment from blood when allowed to stand in the presence of an anticoagulant. This is increased when cells stack together (form *rouleaux*), and in pregnancy and inflammatory disease. It is decreased by low plasma fibrinogen. Erythrocytes have a normal volume of 85 fl (85×10^{-15}/L; mean cell volume, MCV), and ~30 pg of haemoglobin (30×10^{-12}/g; mean cell haemoglobin, MCH). The mean cell haemoglobin concentration (MCHC) is thus ~350 g/L. Blood contains ~160 g (male) and ~140 g (female) of haemoglobin per litre. Erythrocytes have an average lifespan of 120 days. Their formation (erythropoiesis) and erythrocyte-related diseases are discussed in Chapter 6.

$$MCV = \frac{PCV}{RCC}; \quad MCH = \frac{Hb}{RCC}; \quad MCHC = \frac{MCH}{MCV} \text{ or } \frac{Hb}{PCV}$$

Leucocytes (white cells)

Leucocytes defend the body against infection by foreign material. The normal total count in adults is $4–11 \times 10^9$/L, although considerable variations occur. In the newborn the count is ~20×10^9/L. Three main types are present in blood: **granulocytes**, **lymphocytes** and **monocytes**. Granulocytes are further classified as **neutrophils**, containing neutral-staining granules, **eosinophils**, containing acid-staining granules, and **basophils**, containing basic-staining granules. All are involved in the inflammatory response and release inflammatory mediators.

Neutrophils migrate to areas of infection (**chemotaxis**) and destroy bacteria by **phagocytosis**. They have a very short half-life of ~6 h. Eosinophils are less motile than neutrophils and are effective against larger parasites. They are increased in allergic diseases. Basophils contain histamine and heparin and are similar to tissue **mast** cells.

Lymphocytes originate in the marrow but mature in the lymph nodes, thymus and spleen before returning to the circulation. Most remain in the lymphatic system. They are critical components of the **immune** system and produce immunoglobulins (antibodies).

Monocytes have a clear cytoplasm and are larger than granulocytes. After formation in the marrow they circulate in the blood for ~72 h before entering the tissues and becoming **macrophages**, to form the **reticulo-endothelial system** in the liver, spleen and lymph nodes.

Platelets

Platelets are small (~3 μm) vesicle-like structures formed from **megakaryocytes** in the bone marrow. They contain dense granules, microtubules and lyosomes, and have membrane receptors for ADP and collagen. The granules contain serotonin (5-HT) and ADP. They play an important role in **haemostasis** (see Chapter 7). Platelets have a lifespan of ~4 days.

6 Erythropoiesis, haemoglobin and anaemia

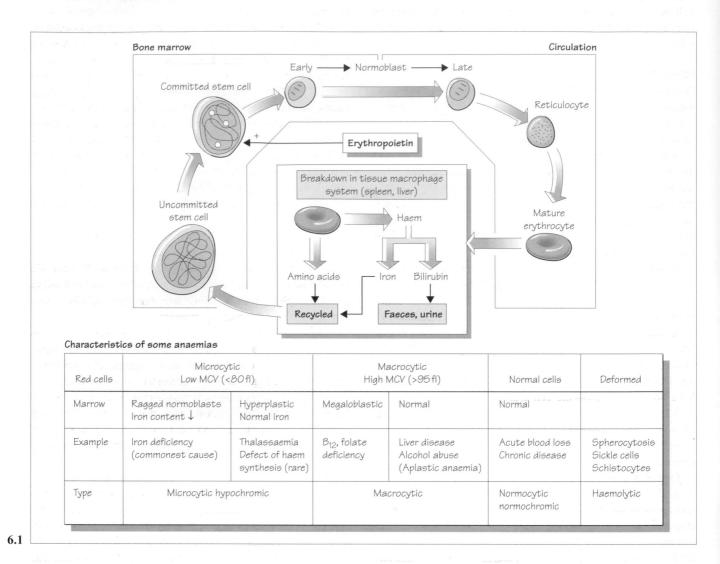

6.1

Characteristics of some anaemias

Red cells	Microcytic Low MCV (<80 fl)		Macrocytic High MCV (>95 fl)		Normal cells	Deformed
Marrow	Ragged normoblasts Iron content ↓	Hyperplastic Normal iron	Megaloblastic	Normal	Normal	
Example	Iron deficiency (commonest cause)	Thalassaemia Defect of haem synthesis (rare)	B₁₂, folate deficiency	Liver disease Alcohol abuse (Aplastic anaemia)	Acute blood loss Chronic disease	Spherocytosis Sickle cells Schistocytes
Type	Microcytic hypochromic		Macrocytic		Normocytic normochromic	Haemolytic

Erythropoiesis leads to the formation of new red blood cells (**erythrocytes**). **Anaemia** is any condition in which there is a reduced blood haemoglobin, resulting in impaired ability of the blood to transport O_2. Some anaemias are associated with abnormal haemoglobins.

Erythropoiesis

Erythrocytes originate from **committed stem cells** in the bone marrow of the adult, and liver and spleen of the fetus. Damage to the marrow can result in erythropoiesis from the liver and spleen of adults. Committed stem cells differentiate into **erythroblasts (early normoblasts)**, which are relatively large (~15 μm) and nucleated. As differentiation proceeds the cells shrink, haemoglobin is synthesized, and in the **late normoblast** the nucleus breaks up and disappears. The young erythrocyte shows a reticulum on staining, and is called a **reticulocyte**. As it ages, the reticulum disappears and the characteristic biconcave

shape develops. Normally 1–2% of circulating red cells are reticulocytes. This increases when erythropoiesis is enhanced, for example by increased **erythropoietin**. About 2×10^{11} erythrocytes are produced from the marrow each day.

Erythropoietin is a glycoprotein hormone produced mainly by the kidneys in adults. In the fetus the main source is the liver. Erythropoietin increases the number of committed stem cells and promotes the production of erythrocytes. The key stimulus for increased erythropoietin is hypoxia. Altitude and chronic respiratory diseases cause the P_{O_2} of the blood to fall, and there is a greatly increased number of erythrocytes (**polycythaemia**) and haematocrit. In kidney disease, chronic inflammation and cirrhosis of the liver erythropoietin levels can fall, resulting in anaemia.

Erythrocytes are destroyed by **macrophages** in the liver and spleen after ~120 days. The spleen also sequesters and eradicates defective erythrocytes. The haem group is split from haemoglobin and converted to **biliverdin** and then **bilirubin**.

The iron is conserved and recycled via **transferrin**, an iron transport protein, or stored in **ferritin**. Bilirubin is a brown/yellow compound which is excreted in the bile. An increased rate of haemoglobin breakdown results in excess bilirubin, which stains the tissues (**jaundice**).

Haemoglobin

Haemoglobin has four subunits, each containing a polypeptide **globin** chain and an iron-containing porphyrin, **haem**. Haem is synthesized from succinic acid and glycine, and contains one atom of iron in the **ferrous** state (Fe^{2+}). One molecule of haemoglobin has therefore four atoms of iron, and binds four molecules of O_2. There are several types of haemoglobin, relating to the globin chains. The haem moiety is unchanged. Adult haemoglobin (Hb A) has two α and two β chains. Fetal haemoglobin (Hb F) has two γ chains in place of the β chains, and a high affinity for O_2. There are several **haemoglobinopathies** due to abnormal haemoglobins.

Sickle cell anaemia is the most important and occurs in 10% of the black population. It is caused by substitution of one glutamic acid by valine in the β chain; this haemoglobin is called Hb S. At a low Po_2 Hb S gels, causing deformation (*sickling*) of the erythrocyte. The cell is less flexible and prone to fragmentation, and there is an increased rate of erythrocyte breakdown by macrophages. The Hb S variant is inherited in a Mendelian fashion. Heterozygous offspring with less than 40% HB S normally have no symptoms (**sickle cell trait**). Homozygous offspring with more than 70% HB S develop full **sickle cell anaemia**. There are acute episodes of pain relating to blockage of blood vessels, congestion of the liver and spleen with red cells, and commonly leg ulcers.

Thalassaemia is caused by a defect in synthesis of either the α- or β-globin chains. Several genes are involved. In β thalassaemia there are either fewer or no β chains available. The α chains therefore bind to γ (Hb F) or δ chains (Hb A$_2$). Thalassaemia major (severe β thalassaemia) has high levels of Hb A$_2$ and Hb F, and severe anaemia. The liver and spleen are enlarged and bone expansion causes typical features. Regular transfusions are required, leading to iron overload. In heterozygous β thalassaemia minor there are no symptoms, although HB A$_2$ is elevated and erythrocytes are **microcytic** and **hypochromic**, i.e. **mean cell volume** (MCV), **mean cell haemoglobin content** (MCH) and **mean cell haemoglobin concentration** (MCHC) are reduced. In α **thalassaemia** there are fewer or no α chains. In the latter case the haem binds four γ chains (Hb Barts), and does not bind O_2. Infants have huge spleens and livers and oedema (**hydrops fetalis**), and do not survive. When some α chains are present, patients surviving as adults may produce some Hb H (four β chains); this precipitates in the red cells which are then destroyed in the spleen, and this is therefore enlarged.

Anaemia

Some anaemias result from simple blood loss (haemorrhage, heavy menstruation) or chronic disease (e.g. infection, tumours, renal failure). When the cells have an otherwise normal MCV and MCH (see Chapter 5), the condition is termed **normocytic normochromic** anaemia.

Aplastic anaemia results from an aplastic (nonfunctional) bone marrow and causes **pancytopenia** (reduced red, white and platelet cell count). It is dangerous but uncommon. It can be caused by certain chemicals and drugs (particularly anticancer drugs), radiation, infections (e.g. viral hepatitis, TB) and pregnancy, where it has a 90% mortality. There is a rare inherited condition, **Fanconi's anaemia** which gives rise to a defect in stem cell production and differentiation. Clinical signs include anaemia, bleeding and infections. The condition is variable, and can show either spontaneous remission or gradual and persistent deterioration. Transfusions can be used for maintenance, but long-term treatment may require a bone marrow transplant.

Haemolytic anaemia results from an excessive rate of erythrocyte destruction, and thus causes jaundice. It is associated with blood transfusion mismatch, **haemolytic anaemia of the newborn** (see Chapter 8), abnormal erythrocyte fragility and haemoglobins, and several other disorders including auto-immune, liver and hereditary diseases.

In **hereditary haemolytic anaemia** (familial spherocytosis) erythrocytes have a more spheroid appearance, are more fragile, and are more rapidly destroyed in the spleen. It is relatively common, affecting 1 in 5000 Caucasians. Jaundice is common but not invariable at birth, and may appear after several years. Patients may develop aplastic anaemia after infections, and **megaloblastic anaemia** from folate deficiency as a result of high bone marrow activity. Removal of the spleen is normally recommended.

Megaloblastic anaemia. Maturation of the normoblast requires **vitamin B$_{12}$** (cyanocobalamin) and **folate**, which is commonly given in pregnancy with iron. A reduction in vitamin B$_{12}$ or folate leads to the formation of unusually large normoblasts (**megaloblasts**), which mature as **macrocytes**. These have a large MCV and MCH, although MCHC is normal. The number of red cells is greatly reduced, and the rate of destruction increased. **Folate deficiency** is mostly related to poor diet, in particular in the old or poor. Alcoholism also impairs utilization. Certain anticonvulsant drugs (e.g. phenytoin) have an antifolate action. **Pernicious anaemia** is caused by vitamin B$_{12}$ deficiency as there is defective absorption from the gut. B$_{12}$ is transported across the ileum as a complex with **intrinsic factor**, which is produced by the gastric mucosa. Damage to the gastric mucosa results in pernicious anaemia. B$_{12}$ deficiency can also occur in strict vegans.

Iron deficiency. The daily requirement for **iron** in the diet is small, as the body has an efficient recycling system. It is increased when there is significant blood loss. As a result of menstrual blood loss women have a higher requirement for dietary iron than men. This is increased during pregnancy. **Iron deficiency** causes defective haemoglobin formation and a **microcytic hypochromic** anaemia.

7 Haemostasis and thrombosis

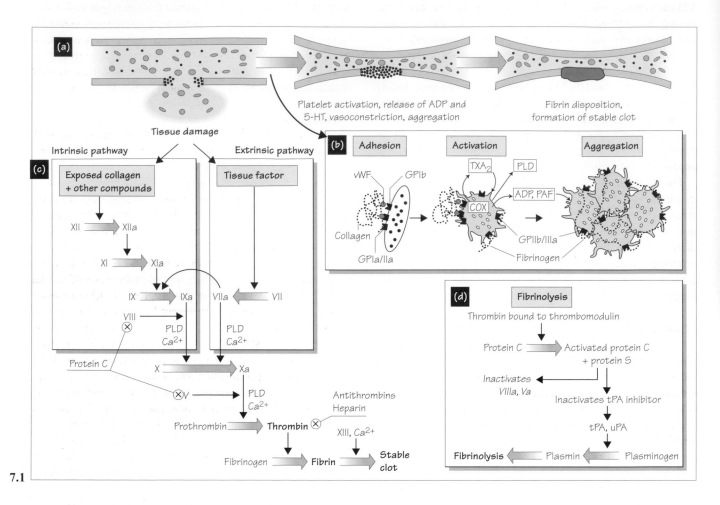

7.1

Haemostasis
Initial response
Damage to blood vessels exposes subendothelial collagen and other macromolecules, to which platelets stick. Platelet **adhesion** is mediated by collagen-bound **von Willebrand factor (vWF)** binding to platelet **GPIb** (glycoprotein) receptors, and direct binding of collagen to **GPIa/IIa** receptors. Adhesion initiates **activation**—platelets change shape, put out pseudopodia and become sticky, and thromboxane A$_2$ (**TXA$_2$**) is synthesized by cyclooxygenase (**COX**). TXA$_2$ causes release of **dense granules** containing **serotonin** (5-HT), **ADP**, platelet activating factor (**PAF**) and **phospholipids** (PLD). TXA$_2$ and 5-HT are powerful vasoconstrictors, and local vessels constrict, reducing flow to the injured area (Fig. 7.1a). If a clot is prevented from forming (by wiping every 15 s), the period before flow stops is a measure of the effectiveness of this initial response (**bleeding time**), and is normally 2–6 min.

Formation of the blood clot
Released ADP and PAF cause activation of further platelets,

exposing GPIIb/IIIa receptors that bind **fibrinogen** and vWF, and as a result platelets rapidly **aggregate** to form a soft **platelet plug** that inhibits further blood loss (Fig. 7.1b). This is then reinforced with **fibrin**, which traps platelets and blood cells. A complex **cascade** of factors is required for fibrin deposition (Fig. 7.1c).

Deposition of fibrin
Fibrinogen is cleaved by **thrombin** (factor IIa), a protease, to sticky and insoluble **fibrin monomers**. In the presence of **factor XIII** and **Ca^{2+}** the monomers polymerize, creating a **stable clot**. Retraction of platelet pseudopodia subsequently causes the clot to contract to ~40% of its original size, becoming tougher and more elastic. Retraction assists repair by drawing the edges of the wound together.

Activation of thrombin
Thrombin is not present in plasma, but is produced when **prothrombin** is activated by **factor X**. This requires **Ca^{2+}**, **factor V** and platelet-derived PLD. Two pathways lead to activation of

factor X. In the **extrinsic pathway**, damaged tissues release **tissue factor** (thromboplastin), which when combined with **factor VIIa** activates factor X. The time taken for clotting to occur following the addition of tissue factor to plasma (fibrinogen and Ca^{2+} in excess) is the **prothrombin time**, and is normally ~14 s. Prothrombin time is prolonged when prothrombin or factors V, VII and X are deficient. The **intrinsic pathway** takes minutes for completion. **Factor XII** is activated by exposed macromolecules following tissue damage, and *in vitro* by negative charges (e.g. glass). A cascade results in activation of factor X, which requires Ca^{2+} and PLD (Fig. 7.1c). Note that thrombin is itself a powerful platelet activator, and also amplifies its own production by activation of factors V, VIII and XI.

The **clotting cascade** is an amplifier. A small stimulus results in a large amount of fibrin. The initial processes take minutes, whereas activation of thrombin and subsequent fibrin deposition is over in seconds. Thus, when blood is placed in glass, there is a delay of 5–10 min before the clot suddenly forms (**clotting time**). Formation of the clot all at once is important for haemostasis. In **haemophilia** the clot forms slowly, and is ineffective.

Inhibitors of clotting and dissolution of the clot

It is important that clots do not form inappropriately. **Prostacyclin** (PGI_2) and nitric oxide are produced by undamaged endothelium and impede platelet adhesion and activation; this helps confine the haemostatic response. Circulating protease inhibitors (**antithrombins**) inhibit thrombin and other factors. **Heparin** is a polysaccharide derived from **mast cells**, and combined with **antithrombin III** is a powerful thrombin inhibitor; *heparan sulphate* on endothelial cells has a similar function. Endothelial cells express **thrombomodulin**, which binds thrombin; this complex activates **protein C**, which with its cofactor **protein S** inactivates factors V and VIII (Fig. 7.1d).

The clot is destroyed by the breakdown of fibrin (**fibrinolysis**) by **plasmin**. This is formed from fibrin-bound **plasminogen** by **tPA, tissue plasminogen activator**, which is released from damaged tissue and endothelium. Thrombin and **urokinase** (uPA) can also cleave plasminogen. Protein C inactivates an inhibitor of tPA, and so promotes fibrinolysis (Fig 7.1d). Fibrinolysis is slower than clotting.

Defects in haemostasis

There are several hereditary **haemophilias** caused by lack of clotting factors. **Clotting time** is prolonged, but **bleeding time** is normal. The most common is **haemophilia A**, a deficiency of factor VIII sex linked to males. **Christmas disease** is a deficiency in factor IX. **Vitamin K** is required by the liver for the production of prothrombin and factors VII, IX and X. It is obtained from intestinal bacteria and food, and disorders of fat absorption or the liver can result in vitamin K deficiency and defective clotting. Prothrombin time is prolonged. **Purpura** is associated with easy bruising and spontaneous haemorrhages in the skin and mucous membranes. It is caused by defective haemostatic vasoconstriction, and the bleeding time is prolonged. Some types of purpura are associated with a reduced platelet production (**thrombocytopenia**). The clotting time may be only slightly prolonged, but the clot is soft and does not retract.

Thrombosis

Thrombosis is inappropriate activation of haemostasis with formation of clots (**thrombi**) inside blood vessels. Three main factors (**Virchow's triad**) predispose to thrombosis. They are: (i) *damage to the endothelium*; (ii) *poor or turbulent blood flow*; and (iii) *hypercoagulability*. (i) is the most important cause for arterial clots, whereas (ii) and (iii) are more important for venous clots. Damage to the endothelium can lead to clot formation in the absence of other factors. **Myocardial infarction** and valve disease often lead to **endocardial damage**, and are associated with a high risk of thrombosis. A major cause of arterial thrombosis is atherosclerosis, and rupture of **atheromatous plaques** (see Chapter 41). Turbulent blood flow or haemodynamic stress (e.g. hypertension) can cause endothelial injury. Poor blood flow (**stasis**) is a major cause of thrombosis in the venous circulation (e.g. deep vein thrombosis, **DVT**), and in the **atrium** following atrioventricular valve stenosis (see Chapter 49). Stasis allows platelets to contact the vessel wall, and activated clotting factors can accumulate because they are not washed away by fresh blood. It also allows unimpeded formation of thrombi. Thrombi can fragment and be carried in the blood as an **embolus**; if this lodges downstream it can cause infarction. A principal danger of venous thrombi is **pulmonary embolism**, a major cause of death.

Hypercoagulability occurs in several genetic and acquired diseases. A high platelet count (**thrombocytosis**) will increase the likelihood of thrombosis. Thrombosis can also result from a defect in factor V (**Leiden's mutation**) that prevents its inactivation by protein C. This is a risk factor for oral contraceptives. Deficiencies in vitamin K, protein C, protein S and antithrombin III promote thrombosis.

Once formed, a thrombus may be modified. Fibrinolysis causes **dissolution**, whereas accumulation of more fibrin and platelets causes **propagation**. If the thrombus does not dissolve, it may over time be invaded by endothelial and smooth muscle cells, in conjunction with fibrosis (**organization**). Channels may develop through the thrombus (**recanalization**), allowing blood to reflow. The thrombus may eventually be incorporated into the vessel wall.

Drugs affecting haemostasis are of major clinical importance, and are discussed in Chapter 43.

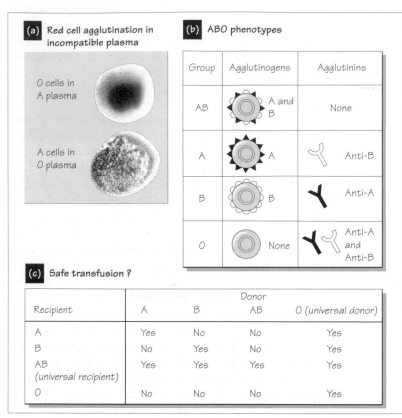

(a) Red cell agglutination in incompatible plasma

O cells in A plasma

A cells in O plasma

(b) ABO phenotypes

Group	Agglutinogens	Agglutinins
AB	A and B	None
A	A	Anti-B
B	B	Anti-A
O	None	Anti-A and Anti-B

(c) Safe transfusion?

	Donor			
Recipient	A	B	AB	O (universal donor)
A	Yes	No	No	Yes
B	No	Yes	No	Yes
AB (universal recipient)	Yes	Yes	Yes	Yes
O	No	No	No	Yes

(d) Relative distribution of ABO blood types by race

Group	Caucasian	Far Eastern	Afro-Caribbean	Native American
A	41%	28%	28%	3%
B	10%	23%	20%	—
AB	4%	13%	5%	—
O	45%	36%	47%	97%

(e) Distribution of Rhesus groups (Caucasians)

Group	Proportion of population	Breakdown of genotypes
RH +	85%	35% DD 48% Dd 2% other + D
RH −	15%	

8.1

Blood groups

If samples of blood from different individuals are mixed together, some combinations result in red cells sticking together as clumps (Fig. 8.1a). This is called **agglutination**, and occurs when the **blood groups** are incompatible. It is caused when antigens (or **agglutinogens**) on the red cell membrane react with specific antibodies (or **agglutinins**) in the plasma. If the quantity (or **titre**) of antibodies is sufficiently high, they bind to their antigens on several red cells and glue the cells together, which then rupture (**haemolyse**). If this occurs following a blood transfusion it can lead to anaemia and other serious complications. The most important blood groups are the **ABO system** and **Rh (Rhesus)** groups.

The ABO system

The ABO system consists of four blood groups: A, B, AB and O. The precise group depends on the presence or absence of two antigens, A and B, on the red cells, and their respective antibodies, α and β, in the plasma (Fig. 8.1b). The A and B antigens on red cells are mostly glycolipids that differ in respect of their terminal sugar. The antigens are also found as glycoproteins in other tissues, including salivary glands, pancreas, lungs and testes, and in saliva and semen.

Group A blood contains the A antigen and β antibody, and group B the B antigen and α antibody. Group AB has both A and B antigens, but neither antibody. Group O blood contains neither antigen, but both α and β antibodies. Group A blood cannot therefore be transfused into people of group B, or vice versa, because antibodies in the recipient react with their respective antigens on the donor red cells and cause agglutination (Fig. 8.1c). As people of group AB have neither α nor β antibodies in the plasma, they can be transfused with blood from any group, and are called **universal recipients**. Group O red cells have neither antigen, and can therefore be transfused into any patient. People of group O are therefore called **universal donors**. Although group O blood contains both antibodies, this can normally be disregarded as they are diluted during transfusion and are bound and neutralized by free A or B antigens in the recipient's plasma. If large or repeated transfusions are required, blood of the same group is used.

Inheritance of ABO blood groups

The expression of A and B antigens is determined genetically. A and B allelomorphs (alternative gene types) are dominant, and O recessive. Therefore AO (**heterozygous**) and AA (**homozygous**) genotypes both have group A phenotypes. An AB genotype produces both antigens, and is thus group AB. The proportion of each blood group varies according to race (Fig. 8.1d), although group O is most common (35–50%). Native Americans are almost exclusively group O.

Rh groups

In ~85% of the population the red cells have a D antigen on the membrane (Fig. 8.1e). Such people are called Rh+ (Rhesus positive), while those who lack the antigen are Rh–. Unlike ABO antigens, the D antigen is not found in other tissues. The antibody to D antigen (**anti-D agglutinin**) is not normally found in the plasma of Rh– individuals, but sensitization and subsequent antibody production occurs if a relatively small amount of Rh+ blood is introduced. This can result from transfusion, or when an Rh– mother has an Rh+ child, and fetal red blood cells enter the maternal circulation during birth. Occasionally fetal cells may cross the placenta earlier in the pregnancy.

Inheritance of Rh groups

The gene corresponding to the D antigen is also called D, and is dominant. When D is absent from the chromosome, its place is taken by the allelomorph of D called d, which is recessive. Individuals who are homozygous and heterozygous for D will be Rh+. About 50% of the population are heterozygous for D, and ~35% homozygous. Blood typing for Rh groups is routinely performed for prospective parents to determine the likelihood of **haemolytic disease** in the offspring.

Haemolytic disease of the newborn

Most pregnancies with Rh– mothers and Rh+ fetuses are normal, but in some cases a severe reaction may occur. Anti-D antibody in the mother's blood can cross the placenta and agglutinate fetal red cells expressing D antigen. The titre of antibody is generally too low to be of consequence during a first pregnancy with a Rh+ fetus, but it can be dangerously increased during subsequent pregnancies, or if the mother was previously sensitized with Rh+ blood. Agglutination of the fetal red cells and consequent haemolysis can result in anaemia and other complications. This is known as **haemolytic disease of the newborn** or **erythroblastosis fetalis**. The haemoglobin released is broken down to bilirubin, which in excess results in **jaundice** (yellow staining of the tissues). If the degree of agglutination and anaemia is severe, the fetus develops severe jaundice and is grossly oedematous (**hydrops fetalis**), and often dies *in utero* or shortly after birth.

Prevention and treatment. In previously unsensitized mothers sensitization can be prevented by treatment with anti-D immunoglobulin after birth. This destroys any fetal Rh+ red cells in the maternal circulation before sensitization of the mother can occur. If haemolytic disease is evident in the fetus or newborn, the Rh+ blood can be replaced by Rh– blood immediately after birth. By the time the newborn has regenerated its own Rh+ red cells, the anti-D antibody from the mother will have been reduced to safe levels. Phototherapy is commonly used for jaundice, as light converts bilirubin to a more rapidly eliminated compound.

Other blood groups

Although there are other blood groups, these are of little clinical importance, as humans rarely develop antibodies to the respective antigens. They may, however, be of importance in medicolegal situations, e.g. determination of paternity. An example is the MN group, which is a product of two genes (M and N). A person can therefore be MM, MN or NN, each genome coming from one parent. As with the other groups, analysis of the respective parties' genomes can only determine that the man is *not* the father. This method has been largely superceded by DNA profiling.

Effects of mismatched blood transfusions

When the recipient of a blood transfusion has a significant plasma titre of α, β or anti-D antibodies, donor red cells expressing the respective antigen will rapidly agglutinate and haemolyse (**haemolytic transfusion reaction**). If the subsequent accumulation of bilirubin is sufficiently large, **haemolytic jaundice** develops. In severe cases renal failure may develop. Antibodies in the donor blood are rarely problematical, as they are diluted and removed in the recipient.

Blood storage

Blood is stored for transfusions at 4°C in the presence of an agent that chelates free Ca^{2+} to prevent clotting, for example citrate, oxalate and EDTA (see Chapter 7). Even under these conditions the red cells deteriorate, although they last much longer in the presence of glucose, which provides a metabolic substrate. The cell membrane Na^+ pump works more slowly in the cold, with the result that Na^+ enters the cell, and K^+ leaves. This causes water to move into the cell so that it swells, and becomes more spherocytic. On prolonged storage the cells become fragile, and **haemolyse** (fragment) easily. Neither leucocytes nor platelets survive storage well, and disappear within a day of transfusion. Blood banks normally remove all the donor agglutinins (antibodies), although for small transfusions these would be sufficiently diluted to be of no threat. Great care is now taken to screen potential donors for blood-borne diseases (e.g. hepatitis, HIV).

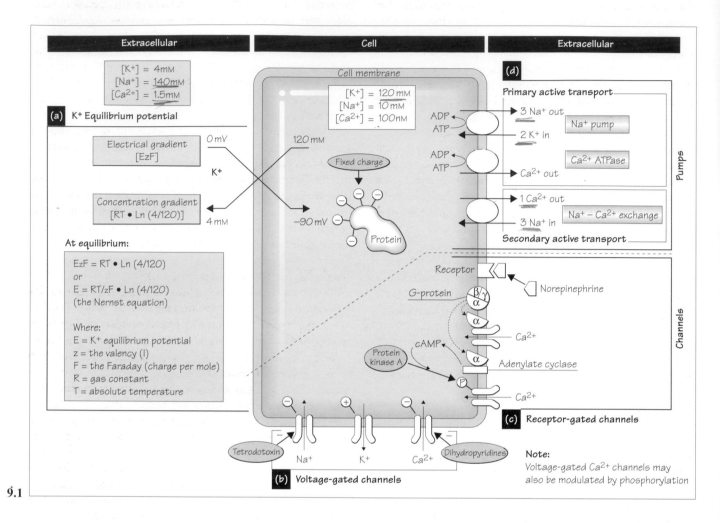

9.1

The cell membrane is composed of a lipid bilayer that has an intrinsically low permeability to charged ions. Spanning the bilayer, however, are a variety of structures through which ions can enter or leave the cell. **Ion channels** allow specific ions to move **passively**, as though through a pore. By contrast, **ion pumps** use energy to **actively transport** ions across the membrane, normally *against* the concentration gradient. Ion channels and pumps are fundamental to cell function. They regulate the ionic gradients across the cell membrane, and determine membrane potential.

The resting membrane potential

At rest, most active ion channels are of a type selective for K$^+$, so that the membrane is more permeable to K$^+$ than other ions. Membranes with this property are called **semipermeable**. The cell contains large negatively charged molecules (e.g. proteins) that cannot cross the membrane. The presence of fixed negative charges attracts positively charged ions. As the membrane is most permeable to K$^+$, this leads to an accumulation of K$^+$ within the cell. However, the *electrical* forces attracting K$^+$ into the cell are then counterbalanced by the increased *concentration gradient*, which tends to drive K$^+$ out of the cell. An equilibrium is reached when these two opposing forces exactly balance. In cardiac muscle cells this occurs when intracellular [K$^+$] is ~120 mM for an extracellular [K$^+$] of ~4 mM. The opposing effect of the concentration gradient means that slightly fewer positive charges (in this case K$^+$ ions) move into the cell than there are intracellular negative charges (e.g. proteins). The inside of the cell is therefore negatively charged compared to the outside (*charge separation*), and as a result a potential develops across the membrane. If the membrane was only permeable to K$^+$, the potential at equilibrium would be defined entirely by the concentration gradient for K$^+$ across the membrane. This is the **K$^+$ equilibrium potential**, and it can be calculated from the **Nernst equation** (Fig. 9.1a).

The actual **resting membrane potential** (RMP) is less negative than the theoretical K$^+$ equilibrium potential. This is because other ions (e.g. Na$^+$) can also cross the membrane, although the membrane permeability for these ions is much less than that for K+. Unlike K+, Na+ has a concentration gradient that is far from equilibrium, as a result of the activity of the **Na+ pump** (Na+, K+-ATPase). This pumps three Na+ ions out of the cell in exchange for two K+ ions into the cell, using ATP as an energy source. As a result intracellular [Na+] is low (~10 mM), even though extracellular [Na+] is high (~140 mM). The equilibrium potential for Na+ (the potential at which electrical and concentration gradient forces would be exactly balanced) is therefore very positive (> +65 mV).

The RMP in a cardiac muscle cell from a ventricle is approximately −90 mV, close to the K+ equilibrium potential. This attracts Na+ ions into the cell. Whereas this inward electrical attraction is balanced in the case of K+ by the *outward* K+ concentration gradient (see above), the concentration gradient for Na+ is *inward* (high Na+ in extracellular fluid, low Na+ in the cell). Thus both concentration and electrical forces draw Na+ *into* the cell, and the **electrochemical gradient** (the net effect of concentration and electrical forces) is inward. The amount of Na+ actually entering the cell is limited by the low membrane permeability for Na+, and the continuous action of the Na+ pump as it pumps Na+ out. An equivalent situation is apparent for Ca2+, as the Ca2+ concentration gradient at rest is ~1.5 mM outside, ~100 nM inside. The small leak of Na+ into the cell causes an inward **background current (I_b)** and slight depolarization, so that RMP is less negative than predicted from the K+ equilibrium potential.

Ion channels and gating

There are many channel types, each of which tends to be selective for a particular ion. When a channel is open ions will move passively down their electrochemical gradient. As ions are charged, this causes an electrical current (*ionic current*). Positive ions entering the cell cause an **inward current** and depolarization. Conventionally current caused by outward movement of negative charge (e.g. Cl−) is also called inward, as it has the same effect. During excitation in cardiac and smooth muscle cells, channels mediating the influx of Na+ or Ca2+ are opened and the cell depolarizes. The transition of a channel between **closed** and **open** states is called **gating**.

Voltage-gated channels

Voltage-gated channels (VGCs) are gated by membrane potential (Fig. 9.1b). Voltage-gated Na+ and Ca2+ channels are activated by depolarization, and are **time dependent**: once opened, they start to **inactivate** immediately. Inactivated channels do not allow the passage of ions. However, they are not in the *closed* state, as they cannot be reopened. This can only happen once they have moved to the true closed state, which does not occur until the membrane potential returns to resting levels. Thus ion flux through VGCs increases rapidly during depolarization, but then falls off at a rate that depends on how fast that type of channel inactivates.

Receptor-gated channels

Receptor-gated channels (RGCs) open when a hormone or neurotransmitter (e.g. norepinephrine) binds to a receptor (Fig. 9.1c). This may involve direct action via **G-proteins** (*GTP-binding proteins*) or indirect action via second messenger systems such as cyclic AMP. Cyclic AMP phosphorylates channel proteins, and apart from directly gating some RGCs, can also *modify* the function of channels such as voltage-gated Ca2+ channels. Other channel types are gated by *intracellular* factors such as [Ca2+] or [ATP].

Channel activity can both be controlled *by*, and exert an important influence *on*, the membrane potential. An important example is the relationship between membrane potential and voltage-activated Ca2+ channels in cardiac muscle and vascular smooth muscle. Depolarization causes channels to open, allowing Ca2+ to enter the cell and initiate contraction. In cardiac muscle, the initial depolarization is caused by opening of Na+ channels and initiation of an **action potential**.

Ion pumps and exchangers (Fig. 9.1d)

Whereas movement of ions through channels is passive, ion pumps use energy to pump against the electrochemical gradient. They are primarily concerned with the regulation of cytosolic ion concentrations rather than cell signalling. An important example is the Na+ pump. Pumps that use ATP are referred to as **primary active transport** processes, and another example is the Ca2+-ATPase that pumps cytosolic Ca2+ into intracellular stores (see Chapters 11, 12). Several other pumps or exchangers use the Na+ electrochemical gradient (maintained by the Na+ pump) as an energy source, and are referred to as **secondary active transport** processes. Na+ binds to the pump and moves down its electrochemical gradient into the cell, effectively twisting the pump so that ions bound on the inside of the membrane are transported out, rather in the way that a water wheel works. Such secondary transport processes include the **Na+–H+ exchanger**, which removes H+ from the cell and helps to control intracellular pH, and the **Na+–Ca2+ exchanger**, in which three Na+ ions are exchanged for one Ca2+ ion. Inhibitors of the Na+ pump (e.g. **digoxin**) will indirectly inhibit these processes by reducing the Na+ gradient. Pumps are stimulated by the concentrations of their respective ions, although their activity may be modulated by second-messenger-mediated phosphorylation.

Relationship between ion pumps and membrane potential

Some pumps transport unequal amounts of charge across the sarcolemma, e.g. the Na+ pump (3 Na+ to 2 K+) and the Na+–Ca2+ exchanger (3 Na+ to 1 Ca2+). Such pumps cause a small but significant ionic current that can affect the membrane potential, and are therefore called **electrogenic**. Electrogenic pumps will themselves be affected by the membrane potential; this is of particular relevance to the Na+–Ca2+ exchanger during the cardiac muscle action potential (see Chapters 10, 11).

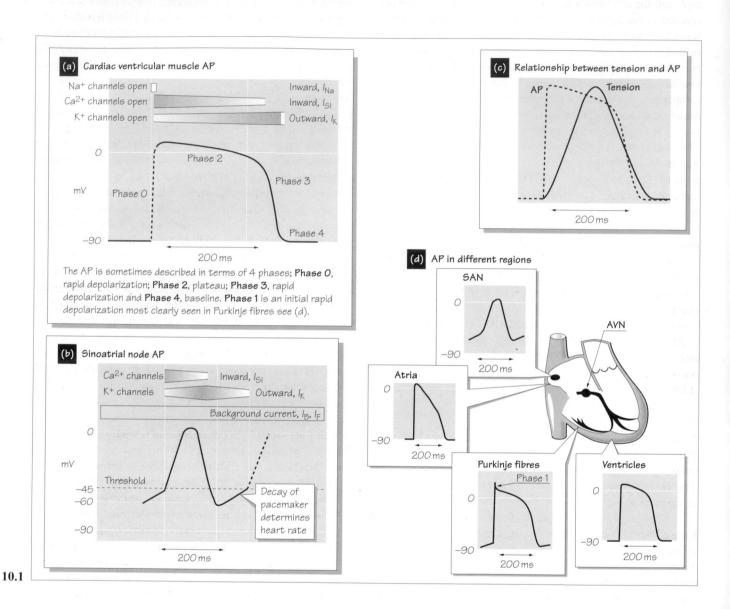

(a) Cardiac ventricular muscle AP

Na⁺ channels open   Inward, I_{Na}
Ca²⁺ channels open   Inward, I_{SI}
K⁺ channels open   Outward, I_K

Phase 2
Phase 3
Phase 0
Phase 4

200 ms

The AP is sometimes described in terms of 4 phases: **Phase 0**, rapid depolarization; **Phase 2**, plateau; **Phase 3**, rapid depolarization and **Phase 4**, baseline. **Phase 1** is an initial rapid depolarization most clearly seen in Purkinje fibres see (d).

(b) Sinoatrial node AP

Ca²⁺ channels   Inward, I_{SI}
K⁺ channels   Outward, I_K
Background current, I_B, I_F

Threshold

Decay of pacemaker determines heart rate

200 ms

(c) Relationship between tension and AP

AP   Tension

200 ms

(d) AP in different regions

SAN
200 ms
AVN
Atria
200 ms
Purkinje fibres
Phase 1
Ventricles
200 ms
200 ms

10.1

An action potential (AP) is the transient depolarization of a cell as a result of activity of ion channels. The cardiac AP is considerably longer than those occurring in nerve or skeletal muscle (~300 ms vs ~1–3 ms). This is due to the presence of a **plateau phase** in cardiac muscle, which lasts for 200–300 ms.

Ventricular muscle action potential (Fig. 10.1a)

Initiation of the action potential

At rest, the membrane is most permeable to K⁺ ions and the **resting potential** is primarily dependent on the K⁺ concentration gradient (see Chapter 9). An AP is initiated when the membrane is depolarized to a **threshold potential** (~–65 mV). The initial depolarization results from transmission from an adjacent cell through **intercalated disks**. At the threshold potential the inward

current caused by entry of Na⁺ through voltage-gated Na⁺ channels (I_{Na}) becomes large enough to overcome the outward current through K⁺ channels, and thus causes further depolarization. This in turn activates more Na⁺ channels. The depolarization thus becomes self generating, and so results in a very rapid upstroke (phase 0; ~500 V/s). At this point the membrane is more permeable to Na⁺ than K⁺ because of the open Na⁺ channels. The Na⁺ concentration gradient therefore becomes the major determinant of membrane potential, and the cell moves *towards* the equilibrium potential for Na⁺ (~+65 mV) (see Chapter 9). It does not reach this potential both because it is limited by the existing K⁺ permeability, and because of rapid **inactivation** (shutting) of the Na⁺ channels. The Na⁺ channels cannot be reactivated until the potential becomes more negative than ~–65 mV. Therefore another AP cannot be initiated until the cell repolarizes *to at least* this potential (**absolute refractory period**). At slightly more negative potentials some Na$^+$ channels reactivate, allowing an AP to be initiated by a sufficiently large stimulus (**relative refractory period**). All Na$^+$ channels are reactivated by the time the cell is completely repolarized. The refractory period, and the length of the AP compared to the twitch (Fig. 10.1c) means that, unlike skeletal muscle, cardiac muscle cannot be tetanized.

The plateau phase
At the end of the upstroke, membrane Na$^+$ permeability returns to its resting value, and in skeletal muscle this results in rapid repolarization. In cardiac muscle, however, the membrane potential decays slowly over ~250 ms before a more rapid repolarization phase. This period of slow decay is the **plateau phase** (phase 2), and is primarily due to Ca^{2+} entering the cell via **voltage-sensitive L-type Ca^{2+} channels**, which activate relatively slowly when the membrane potential becomes more positive than ~–35 mV. The resultant Ca^{2+} current (**slow inward current** or I_{SI}), coupled with a reduced K$^+$ outward current, is sufficient to slow repolarization until the potential falls to ~–20 mV. The length of the plateau is related to slow **inactivation** of Ca^{2+} channels. Ca^{2+} entry during the plateau is vital for contraction; blockers of L-type Ca^{2+} channels (e.g. **dihydropyridines**) reduce force (see Chapter 11).

Repolarization (phase 3)
At the end of the plateau the K$^+$ outward current becomes dominant, and membrane potential returns to its resting level (phase 4). Several types of K$^+$ channel contribute to repolarization. Factors that influence outward current will affect the rate of repolarization, and hence the length of AP.

Role of Na$^+$–Ca^{2+} exchange during the action potential
In the early stages of the plateau, when it is most positive and the Na$^+$ electrochemical gradient is therefore at its smallest, the Na$^+$–Ca^{2+} exchanger may be reversed, and contribute to the inward movement of Ca^{2+}. As the plateau decays and becomes more negative the Na$^+$ electrochemical gradient increases, and the Na$^+$–Ca^{2+} exchanger returns to its usual function of expelling Ca^{2+}. The resulting influx of Na$^+$ ions causes an inward current that may slow repolarization and reduce the rate of decay of the plateau, thus lengthening the AP.

Sinoatrial node and the origin of the heart beat
The AP of the **sinoatrial node** (SAN, Fig. 10.1b) differs in several important aspects from that of the ventricle. The upstroke in the SAN is much slower than in the ventricle. This is because there are no functional Na$^+$ channels, and depolarization is caused by Ca^{2+} entry via slowly activating Ca^{2+} channels. The slower upstroke leads to slower conduction from cell to cell (see Chapter 15). This is of particular importance in the **atrioventricular node** (AVN), which has a similar AP to the SAN.

In direct contrast to the ventricle, the SAN has an unstable resting potential which decays from ~–60 mV to a threshold potential of ~–40 mV, at which point an AP is initiated. The threshold potential is more positive than that in the ventricle, because voltage-gated Ca^{2+} channels, which underlie the upstroke in the SAN, have a more positive threshold than voltage-gated Na$^+$ channels, which underlie the upstroke in the ventricle. The rate of decay of the SAN resting potential determines the rate at which APs are generated, and hence heart rate. The resting potential is therefore commonly called the **pacemaker potential**. The pacemaker potential relies on a K$^+$ outward current that slowly decays with time (I_K), and two relatively stable inward currents, mostly due to the inward movement of Na$^+$. These are I_b, which is also present in other cardiac cells, and I_f ('*funny*'), which appears to be specific to the SAN. As the outward I_K decays, this allows the contribution from the inward I_f and I_b to become more dominant, and the membrane depolarizes.

Factors that influence these currents alter the slope of the pacemaker and thus heart rate, and are called **chronotropic agents**. The sympathetic neurotransmitter norepinephrine increases heart rate by increasing the slope of the pacemaker, caused by an increase in the size of I_f. It also reduces the length of the AP by increasing the rate of Ca^{2+} entry and hence the slope of the upstroke. The parasympathetic transmitter acetylcholine reduces the slope of the pacemaker, and causes a small hyperpolarization, both of which increase the time required to reach threshold, and reduce heart rate.

Action potentials in other regions of the heart (Fig. 10.1d)
AVN APs are similar to those of the SAN. Atrial muscle has a similar AP to ventricular muscle, although the shape is more triangular. **Purkinje fibres** in the conduction system have a spike at the peak of upstroke (phase 1). This relates to a greater inward Na$^+$ current and more rapid upstroke, and contributes to faster conduction. The AVN, bundle of His and Purkinje system may also have decaying resting potentials that can act as pacemakers. However, the SAN is normally fastest and predominates. This is called **dominance** or **overdrive suppression**.

Effects of plasma [K$^+$]
Several conditions increase plasma [K$^+$] (e.g. renal failure, tissue damage). If it rises above ~5.5 mM (**hyperkalaemia**) there can be serious consequences, as the membrane depolarizes and becomes closer to threshold potential. This can cause dangerous arrhythmias, e.g. ventricular fibrillation, especially where the myocardium is diseased (see Chapter 46). Hyperkalaemia also slows and weakens the AP upstroke due to partial inactivation of Na$^+$ channels, and slows conduction. Above 8 mM this leads to complete cessation of conduction (**heart block**). Conversely **hypokalaemia** (< ~3 mM [K$^+$]) hyperpolarizes the membrane, making it more difficult to reach threshold and also affecting conduction. Hypokalaemia is commonly associated with diuretic therapy in heart disease (e.g. Chapter 45).

11 Excitation–contraction coupling in cardiac muscle cells

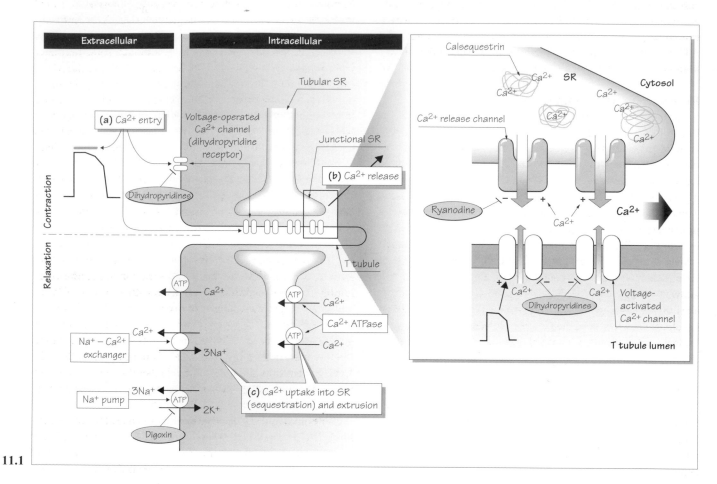

11.1

Cardiac muscle contracts when cytosolic [Ca²⁺] rises above about 100 nM. This rise in [Ca²⁺] couples the action potential (AP) to contraction, and the mechanisms involved are referred to as **excitation–contraction coupling**. The relationship between cardiac muscle force and stretch is discussed in Chapter 14. The ability of cardiac muscle to generate force *for any given fibre length* is described as its **contractility**. This depends on cytosolic [Ca²⁺], and to a lesser extent on factors which affect Ca²⁺ sensitivity of the contractile apparatus. The contractility of cardiac muscle is primarily dependent on the way that the cell handles Ca²⁺.

Initiation of contraction

During the **plateau phase** of the AP, Ca²⁺ enters the cell through L-**type voltage-gated Ca²⁺ channels** in the **sarcolemma** (muscle cell membrane; Fig. 11.1a). L-type channels are specifically blocked by **dihydropyridines** (e.g. **nifedipine**) and *verapamil*. However, the amount of Ca²⁺ that enters the cell is less than 20% of that required for the observed rise in cytosolic [Ca²⁺] ([Ca²⁺]ᵢ). The rest is released from the **sarcoplasmic reticulum** (SR), where Ca²⁺ is stored in high concentrations associated

with **calsequestrin** (Fig. 11.1b). The action potential travels into the **T tubules** and during the first 1–2 ms of the plateau Ca²⁺ enters and causes a rise in [Ca²⁺] in the gap between the sarcolemma and the **junctional SR**. This rise in [Ca²⁺] is sufficient to activate Ca²⁺-sensitive **Ca²⁺ release channels** in the SR, through which stored Ca²⁺ floods into the cytoplasm down its concentration gradient. This process is called **calcium-induced calcium release (CICR)**. The combination of Ca²⁺ release and Ca²⁺ entry across the membrane causes a rapid increase in [Ca²⁺]ᵢ over the next 10 ms, and initiates contraction. Note that cardiac muscle differs from skeletal muscle, in that CICR is entirely responsible for Ca²⁺ release from the SR. The action potential itself in the absence of Ca²⁺ entry cannot cause Ca²⁺ release, and in the *absence of external Ca²⁺ there is no contraction of cardiac muscle*.

The amount of Ca²⁺ released depends both on how much is stored in the SR and on the amount of Ca²⁺ entering across the sarcolemma. Modulation of the latter is a key way in which cardiac function is regulated (see Inotropic agents below). Peak [Ca²⁺]ᵢ normally rises to ~2 μM, although maximum contraction occurs when [Ca²⁺]ᵢ rises above 10 μM.

Generation of tension

The physical arrangement of **actin** and **myosin** filaments is discussed in Chapter 2. Force is generated when the myosin heads protruding from the thick filament bind to sites on actin to form **crossbridges**, and drag the actin past in a ratchet fashion, using ATP bound to myosin as an energy source. This is the **sliding filament** or **crossbridge mechanism** of muscle contraction.

Regulation of crossbridge formation

In cardiac muscle as in skeletal muscle, $[Ca^{2+}]_i$ controls crossbridge formation via the regulatory proteins **tropomyosin** and **troponin**. Tropomyosin is a coiled strand which, at rest, lies in the cleft between the two actin chains that form the thin filament helix, and covers the myosin binding sites on the actin. The myosin heads therefore cannot bind, and there is no tension. Troponin is formed from a complex of three smaller globular proteins (**troponin C, I and T**), which is bound to tropomyosin by **troponin T** at intervals of 40 nm. When $[Ca^{2+}]_i$ rises above 100 nM, Ca^{2+} binds to **troponin C** and there is a conformational change involving dissociation of **troponin I** from actin, which allows tropomyosin to shift out of the actin cleft. The binding sites are uncovered, myosin crossbridges form, and tension develops. Tension is related to the number of active crossbridges, and will increase until all troponin C is bound to Ca^{2+} ($[Ca^{2+}]_i > 10 \mu M$).

Relaxation mechanisms

When $[Ca^{2+}]_i$ rises above the resting level (~100 nM), ATP-dependent Ca^{2+} pumps (**Ca^{2+}-ATPase**) in the tubular part of the SR are activated, and start to pump Ca^{2+} from the cytosol back into the SR (Fig. 11.1c). As the AP repolarizes and voltage-dependent Ca^{2+} channels inactivate, this mechanism reduces $[Ca^{2+}]_i$ towards resting levels, Ca^{2+} ions dissociate from troponin C, and the muscle relaxes.

If there were no other mechanisms to remove Ca^{2+} from the cell, the size of the SR Ca^{2+} store would gradually increase as more Ca^{2+} enters during each AP. Excess Ca^{2+} is transported out of the cell by the **Na^+–Ca^{2+} exchanger** in the sarcolemma (Fig. 11.1c; see Chapter 9). This uses the inward Na^+ electrochemical gradient as an energy source to pump Ca^{2+} out, and in the process three Na^+ ions enter the cell for each Ca^{2+} ion removed. There are also Ca^{2+}-ATPase pumps in the sarcolemma, but their importance is minor. At the end of the AP about 80% of the Ca^{2+} will have been resequestered into the SR, and most of the rest ejected from the cell. The remainder is slowly pumped out during the diastolic interval.

Modulation of cardiac muscle tension

Inotropic agents

Factors that alter the contractility of cardiac muscle are called **inotropic agents.** A positive inotropic agent increases contractility, whereas a negative one decreases it. Most inotropic agents act via mechanisms that regulate $[Ca^{2+}]_i$, although some may alter Ca^{2+} binding to troponin C. For example, a high plasma $[Ca^{2+}]$ increases contractility by increasing Ca^{2+} entry during the AP.

Norepinephrine from sympathetic nerve endings, and to a lesser extent circulating **epinephrine**, are the most important physiological inotropic agents. They also increase heart rate (positive **chronotropes**; see Chapter 10). Norepinephrine binds to β_1-adrenoceptors on the sarcolemma, and thus increases cAMP. cAMP-mediated phosphorylation of Ca^{2+} channels increases Ca^{2+} entry during the AP (see Chapter 9), and thus elevates $[Ca^{2+}]_i$, largely by increasing Ca^{2+} release (see above). Norepinephrine may also activate Ca^{2+} channels directly via G-proteins (see Chapter 9). The rate of Ca^{2+} reuptake into the SR, and hence the rate of relaxation, is also increased by norepinephrine, via cAMP-mediated phosphorylation of **phospholamban**, a regulatory protein associated with the Ca^{2+}-ATPase.

Cardiac glycosides such as **digoxin** are specific inhibitors of the **Na^+ pump** and increase cytosolic $[Na^+]$, so reducing the Na^+ gradient across the sarcolemma that drives Na^+–Ca^{2+} exchange (see Chapter 9). As a result less Ca^{2+} is removed from the cell, and more ends up in the SR. There is therefore more available for release, and peak $[Ca^{2+}]_i$ and tension increases. The clinical use of digoxin is discussed in Chapter 45.

Overstimulation by positive inotropes can lead to **Ca^{2+} overload**, and damage due to excessive uptake of Ca^{2+} by the SR and mitochondria. This is important for the progressive decline in myocardial function seen in **chronic heart failure** (see Chapter 44), when sympathetic stimulation is high.

Acidosis is *negatively* inotropic, largely by interfering with the actions of Ca^{2+}. This is important in **myocardial ischaemia** and **heart failure** (see Chapter 44), where poor perfusion can lead to **lactic acidosis** and so further depress cardiac function.

The influence of heart rate

When heart rate increases there is a proportional rise in cardiac muscle force. This phenomenon is known as the **staircase**, **Treppe** or **Bowditch** effect. It can be attributed both to an increase in cytosolic $[Na^+]$ due to the greater frequency of APs, with a consequent inhibition of the Na^+–Ca^{2+} exchanger (see above), and to a decreased diastolic interval over which Ca^{2+} can be extruded from the cell, resulting in more Ca^{2+} in the SR.

12 Vascular smooth muscle excitation–contraction coupling

12.1

Vascular smooth muscle (VSM) contraction is, like that of cardiac muscle, controlled by the *intracellular Ca²⁺ concentration* $[Ca^{2+}]_i$. Unlike cardiac muscle cells, however, VSM cells lack troponin and utilize a *myosin-based system* to regulate contraction.

Regulation of contraction by Ca²⁺ and myosin phosphorylation

Vasoconstricting stimuli initiate VSM cell contraction by increasing $[Ca^{2+}]_i$ from its basal level of ~100 nM. Force development is proportional to the increase in $[Ca^{2+}]_i$, with maximal contraction occurring at ~1 μM $[Ca^{2+}]_i$. The rise in $[Ca^{2+}]_i$ promotes its binding to the cytoplasmic regulatory protein **calmodulin**. Once a calmodulin molecule has bound four Ca²⁺ ions, it can activate the enzyme **myosin light-chain kinase** (MLCK). MLCK in turn phosphorylates two 20-kDa subunits ('**light chains**') contained within the 'head' of each myosin molecule. Phosphorylated myosin then forms crossbridges with actin, using ATP hydrolysis as an energy source to produce contraction. Actin–myosin interactions during crossbridge cycling are similar to those in cardiac myocytes (see Chapter 11).

The degree of myosin light-chain phosphorylation, which determines crossbridge turnover, is a balance between the activity of MLCK and a **myosin light-chain phosphatase** which dephosphorylates the light chains. Once $[Ca^{2+}]_i$ falls, MLCK activity diminishes and relaxation occurs as light-chain phosphorylation is returned to basal levels by the phosphatase.

VSM cells *in vivo* maintain a tonic level of partial contraction that varies with fluctuations in the vasoconstricting and vasodilating influences to which they are exposed. VSM cells avoid fatigue during prolonged contractions because their rate of ATP consumption is 300-fold lower than that of skeletal muscle fibres. This is possible because the crossbridge cycle is much slower than in striated muscles. The maximum crossbridge cycling rate of smooth muscle during shortening is only about 1/10 of that in striated muscles, as a result of differences in the types of myosin present. In addition, once they have shortened, vascular cells can maintain contraction with an even lower expenditure of ATP because the myosin crossbridges remain attached to actin for a longer time, thus 'locking in' shortening.

Vasoconstricting mechanisms

The binding to receptors of **norepinephrine** and other important vasoconstrictors such as **endothelin, thromboxane A$_2$, angiotensin II** and **vasopressin** stimulates VSM contraction via common **G-protein-mediated** pathways (Fig. 12.1a).

Ca^{2+} release

Binding of vasoconstrictors to receptors activates the G-protein **Gq**, which stimulates the enzyme **phospholipase C**. Phospholipase C splits the membrane phospholipid phosphatidylinositol 1,4-bisphosphate, generating the second messengers inositol 1,4,5-triphosphate (**IP$_3$**), and diacylglycerol (**DAG**). IP$_3$ binds to and opens Ca^{2+} channels on the membrane of the **sarcoplasmic reticulum** (SR). This allows Ca^{2+}, which is stored in high concentrations within the SR, to flood out into the cytoplasm and rapidly increase [Ca^{2+}]$_i$. DAG activates **protein kinase C** (PKC).

Effects on ion channels

Vasoconstrictors also cause **membrane depolarization** via several mechanisms. First, the release of SR Ca^{2+} which they initiate opens **Ca^{2+}-activated chloride channels** in the plasma membrane. Second, vasoconstrictors may cause depolarization by *inhibiting* the activity of **K$^+$ channels**. Third, vasoconstrictors induce both membrane depolarization and Ca^{2+} entry into VSM cells by opening **receptor-gated cation channels**, which allow the influx of both Na$^+$ and Ca^{2+} ions.

The membrane depolarization elicited by vasoconstrictors opens **voltage-gated Ca^{2+} channels** similar to those found in cardiac myocytes. With sufficient depolarization, some blood vessels may fire brief Ca^{2+} channel-mediated APs that cause transient contractions. More often, however, blood vessels respond to vasoconstrictors with graded depolarizations, during which sufficient Ca^{2+} influx occurs to cause more sustained contractions.

There is recent evidence that vasoconstrictors can promote Ca^{2+} influx by two additional mechanisms related to pathways described above. First, depletion of Ca^{2+} from the SR due to the action of IP$_3$ opens a **store-operated Ca^{2+} channel** in the cell membrane which admits Ca^{2+} to the cell. Second, G-protein-linked mechanisms directly enhance the opening of voltage-gated Ca^{2+} channels, probably via channel phosphorylation.

As well as raising [Ca^{2+}]$_i$, vasoconstrictors also promote contraction by a process termed **Ca^{2+} sensitization**. Ca^{2+} sensitization is caused by the inhibition of myosin phosphatase. This increases myosin light-chain phosphorylation, and therefore force development, even with minimal increases in [Ca^{2+}]$_i$ and MLCK activity. Recent evidence suggests that phosphatase inhibition may be primarily caused by **rhoA kinase**, an enzyme stimulated by the *ras* type G-protein **rhoA**, which is activated by vasoconstrictors. PKC may also contribute to Ca^{2+} sensitization.

The relative importance of the excitatory mechanisms listed above varies between different vasoconstrictors and vascular beds. In resistance arteries depolarization and Ca^{2+} influx through voltage-gated channels are probably most important.

Ca^{2+} removal mechanisms

Several mechanisms serve to remove Ca^{2+} from the cytoplasm. These are continually active, allowing cells both to recover from stimulation and to maintain a low basal [Ca^{2+}]$_i$ in the face of the enormous electrochemical gradient tending to drive Ca^{2+} into cells even when they are not stimulated. The **smooth endoplasmic reticulum Ca^{2+}-ATPase (SERCA)** pumps Ca^{2+} from the cytoplasm into the SR. This process is referred to as **Ca^{2+} sequestration**. A similar **plasma membrane Ca^{2+}-ATPase (PMCA)** pumps Ca^{2+} from the cytoplasm into the extracellular space (**Ca^{2+} extrusion**). Cells also extrude Ca^{2+} via a **Na/Ca antiport** located in the cell membrane, which is similar to that found in cardiac cells (see Chapter 11). The Na/Ca antiport may be localized to areas of the plasma membrane which are approached closely by the sarcoplasmic reticulum, allowing any Ca^{2+} leaking from the SR to be quickly ejected from the cell without causing tension development.

Vasodilator mechanisms

Most vasodilators acting on smooth muscle cells cause relaxation by activating either the cyclic **GMP** (e.g. nitric oxide, ANP) or cyclic **AMP** (e.g. adenosine, prostacyclin, β-receptor agonists) second messenger systems (Fig. 12.1b). Both second messengers activate kinases, which act by phosphorylating overlapping sets of cellular proteins. cGMP activates **cyclic GMP-dependent protein kinase (PKG)**. The mechanisms by which PKG causes relaxation have not been conclusively established. It has been reported, however, that PKG causes hyperpolarization by activating K$^+$ channels, and that it stimulates both Ca^{2+} sequestration and extrusion by activating the SERCA and PMCA.

Cyclic AMP exerts its effects via **cyclic AMP-dependent protein kinase (protein kinase A or PKA)**, although high levels of cAMP have also been shown to stimulate PKG. PKA is thought to cause smooth muscle cell relaxation by lowering [Ca^{2+}]$_i$. There is evidence that it does so by stimulating the SERCA, and also by opening **ATP-sensitive (K$_{ATP}$)** and **Ca^{2+}-activated K$^+$ (BK) channels**. This causes membrane hyperpolarization, which inhibits Ca^{2+} influx by switching off voltage-gated Ca^{2+} channels, a fraction of which are open even at the resting membrane potential. Hyperpolarization is additionally reported to inhibit phospholipase C activity, thereby reducing IP$_3$ production. PKA can also phosphorylate MLCK, thereby inhibiting its activity. The contribution of this mechanism to relaxation under physiological conditions is, however, controversial.

13 Cardiac cycle

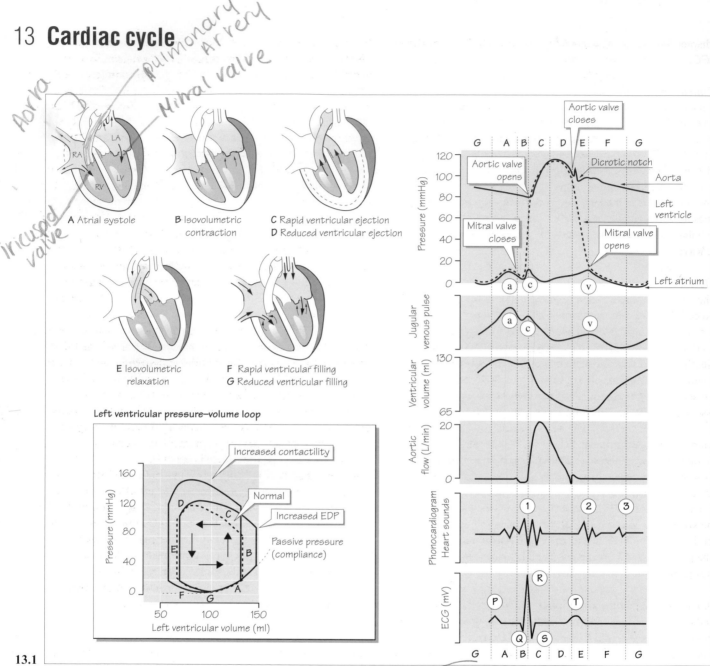

Aorta
pulmonary Artery
Mitral valve
Tricuspid valve

A Atrial systole   **B** Isovolumetric contraction   **C** Rapid ventricular ejection / **D** Reduced ventricular ejection

E Isovolumetric relaxation   **F** Rapid ventricular filling / **G** Reduced ventricular filling

Left ventricular pressure–volume loop

Increased contactility
Normal
Increased EDP
Passive pressure (compliance)

Aortic valve closes
Aortic valve opens
Dicrotic notch
Aorta
Left ventricle
Mitral valve closes
Mitral valve opens
Left atrium

13.1

The **cardiac cycle** is the sequence of mechanical events that occurs during a single heart beat.

Towards the end of **diastole** (G) all chambers of the heart are relaxed. The valves between the atria and ventricles are open (**AV valves**: right, **tricuspid**; left, **mitral**), because atrial pressure remains slightly greater than ventricular pressure until the ventricles are fully distended. The **pulmonary** and **aortic** (semilunar) **outflow valves** are closed, as pulmonary artery and aortic pressure is greater than ventricular pressure. The cycle begins when the **sinoatrial node** initiates the heart beat.

Atrial systole (A)
Contraction of the atria completes ventricular filling. At rest,

the atria contribute less than 20% of final ventricular volume. The remainder is contributed by venous pressure. The atrial contribution increases as heart rate rises, as diastole shortens and there is less time for ventricular filling. There are no valves between the veins and atria, and some blood regurgitates into the veins. The **a wave** of atrial and venous pressure traces reflects atrial systole. Ventricular volume after filling is known as **end-diastolic volume** (EDV), and is ~120–140 ml. The equivalent pressure (**end-diastolic pressure**, EDP) is less than 10 mmHg, and is higher in the left ventricle than in the right due to the more muscular and therefore stiffer left ventricular wall. EDV is an important determinant of the strength of the subsequent contraction (Starling's Law, see

Chapter 14). Atrial depolarization causes the **P wave** of the ECG.

Ventricular systole

Ventricular contraction causes a sharp rise in ventricular pressure, and the atrioventricular (AV) valves close once this exceeds atrial pressure. Ventricular depolarization is associated with the **QRS complex** of the ECG. During the initial phase of ventricular contraction pressure is less than that in the pulmonary artery and aorta, so the outflow valves remain closed. This is **isovolumetric contraction** (B), as ventricular volume does not change. The increasing pressure causes the AV valves to bulge into the atria, resulting in the small atrial pressure wave (**c wave**).

Ejection

The outflow valves open when pressure in the ventricle exceeds that in the artery. Note that pulmonary artery pressure (~15 mmHg) is considerably less than that in the aorta (~80 mmHg). Flow into the arteries is initially very rapid (**rapid ejection phase**, C), but as contraction wanes ejection is reduced (**reduced ejection phase**, D). Active contraction ceases during the second half of ejection, and the muscle repolarizes. This is associated with the **T wave** of the ECG. Ventricular pressure during the reduced ejection phase is slightly less than that in the artery, but blood continues to flow out of the ventricle because of momentum. Eventually the flow briefly reverses, causing closure of the outflow valve and a small increase in aortic pressure, the **dicrotic notch**.

The amount of blood ejected by the ventricle in one beat is the **stroke volume**, ~70 ml. About 50 ml of blood is therefore left in the ventricle at the end of systole (**end-systolic volume**). The proportion of EDV that is ejected (stroke volume/EDV) is the **ejection fraction**.

Diastole—relaxation and refilling

In the period following closure of the outflow valves the ventricles are rapidly relaxing. Ventricular pressure is still greater than atrial pressure however, and the AV valves remain closed. This is known as **isovolumetric relaxation** (E). During the last two-thirds of systole atrial pressure rises as a result of filling from the veins (**v wave**). When ventricular pressure falls below atrial pressure, the AV valves open, and atrial pressure falls as the ventricles rapidly refill (**rapid ventricular refilling**, F). This is assisted by elastic recoil of the ventricular walls, essentially sucking in the blood. As the ventricles relax completely refilling slows (**reduced refilling**, G). This continues during the last two-thirds of diastole due to venous flow. At rest, diastole is twice the length of systole, but decreases proportionately during exercise and as heart rate increases.

The pressure–volume loop

Ventricular pressure plotted against volume generates a loop (Fig. 13.1). The shape of the loop is affected by the **contractility** (see Chapters 11, 14) and **compliance** ('*stretchiness*') of the ventricle, and factors that alter **refilling** or **ejection** (e.g. CVP, afterload). The bottom dotted line shows the passive elastic properties of the ventricle (compliance). If compliance was decreased as a result of fibrotic damage following an infarct, the curve would be steeper. The area of the loop (Δ pressure $\times \Delta$ volume) is a measure of work done by the heart during a beat, and is an indicator of cardiac function. A common clinical estimate of **stroke work** is calculated from mean arterial pressure $\times$ stroke volume.

Cardiac auscultation—heart sounds and murmurs

The **first heart sound** (S_1) is low frequency, and associated with closure of the AV valves. These normally close simultaneously, and **splitting** of S_1 may reflect delayed electrical conduction in the left or right bundles of His (see Chapter 15). The **second heart sound** (S_2) reflects pulmonary and aortic valve closure, and often splits in young people during inspiration and exercise due to a longer ejection period in the right ventricle. The **third heart sound** (S_3) is associated with rapid refilling, and is most commonly heard in young people. In adults it may represent ventricular stiffness or a raised EDP. A **fourth heart sound** (S_4) is associated with atrial systole, but is rarely audible except when EDP is raised. When S_3 and/or S_4 are present, they produce a triple sound similar to a galloping horse, a '**gallop rhythm**' (e.g. heart failure, see Chapter 44).

Cardiac **murmurs** are caused by turbulent bloodflow. A murmur during the ejection phase is often heard in young people, and is benign. Other murmurs can reflect valve defects (see Chapters 49, 50). In **stenosis** the valve is narrowed, and blood velocity increases. This promotes turbulence and creates a murmur. In **incompetence** the valve leaks blood while closed, and this **regurgitation** is heard as a dull roar. Aortic incompetence leads to a diastolic murmur and softening and prolongation of the second heart sound. A **thrill** is a clear vibration.

The arterial pulse

The peripheral pulse is caused by pressure waves travelling down the arterial tree. The shape of the pulse is modified by the compliance and size of the artery. A stiff artery, as in advancing age or atherosclerosis, results in a sharper pulse. The pulse also becomes sharper as artery size decreases. Reflections back up the artery from points where resistance to flow increases, e.g. where the artery divides, can give rise to further peaks. A small, slowly rising pulse can be caused by stenosis of the aortic valve. Aortic valve incompetence can cause a hard knocking sensation as the pulse pressure falls rapidly after each beat. This is called a **collapsing** or **Corrigan** pulse (see Chapter 49).

The **jugular venous pulse** reflects the right atrial pressure, and has corresponding **a, c** and **v waves** (see above).

14 Control of cardiac output and Starling's Law of the Heart

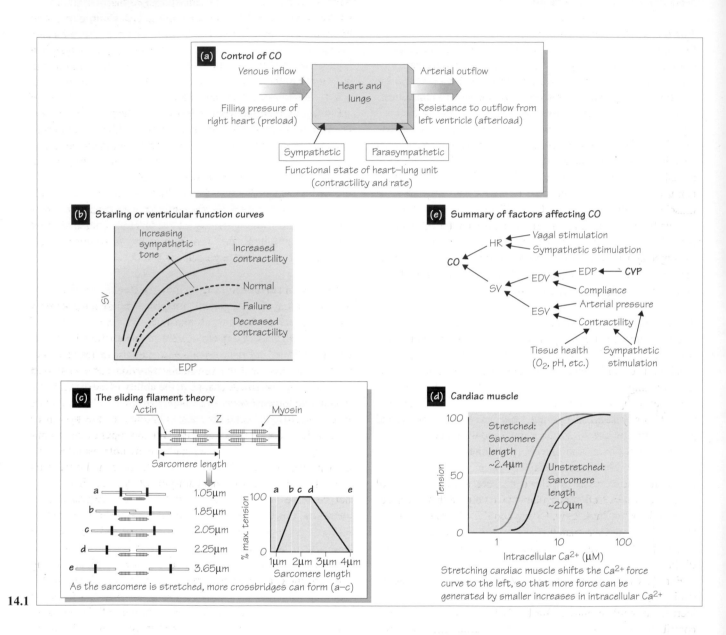

(a) Control of CO

Venous inflow → Heart and lungs → Arterial outflow

Filling pressure of right heart (preload)

Resistance to outflow from left ventricle (afterload)

Sympathetic   Parasympathetic

Functional state of heart–lung unit (contractility and rate)

(b) Starling or ventricular function curves

Increasing sympathetic tone

Increased contractility

Normal

Failure

Decreased contractility

SV / EDP

(e) Summary of factors affecting CO

HR ← Vagal stimulation / Sympathetic stimulation

CO ← HR / SV

EDV ← EDP ← CVP / Compliance

ESV ← Arterial pressure / Contractility

Tissue health (O₂, pH, etc.)   Sympathetic stimulation

(c) The sliding filament theory

Actin   Z   Myosin

Sarcomere length

a   1.05μm
b   1.85μm
c   2.05μm
d   2.25μm
e   3.65μm

a b c d   e

% max. tension 100 / 0

1μm 2μm 3μm 4μm
Sarcomere length

As the sarcomere is stretched, more crossbridges can form (a–c)

(d) Cardiac muscle

Tension 100 / 50 / 0

Stretched: Sarcomere length ~2.4μm

Unstretched: Sarcomere length ~2.0μm

1   10   100
Intracellular Ca²⁺ (μM)

Stretching cardiac muscle shifts the Ca²⁺ force curve to the left, so that more force can be generated by smaller increases in intracellular Ca²⁺

14.1

Cardiac output (CO) is the volume of blood pumped through the heart per minute, i.e. stroke volume (SV) × heart rate (HR). In a normal 70-kg man, cardiac output at rest is about 5 L/min, but during strenuous exercise this can rise to 25 L/min or more.

Control of cardiac output

If the heart and lungs are considered as a unit, it can be seen that only three things can directly influence cardiac output (Fig. 14.1a). These are the filling pressure of the right heart (**preload**), the resistance to outflow from the left ventricle (**afterload**), and the functional state of the heart. The latter includes heart rate and **contractility** (see Chapter 11), which are modulated by the **sympathetic** and **parasympathetic** nervous systems.

Filling pressure and stroke volume

The amount of blood in the ventricle at the start of systole (**end-diastolic volume**, EDV) depends on the **end-diastolic pressure** (EDP) and the **compliance** of the ventricular wall (how easy it is to inflate). Right ventricular EDP is primarily dependent on **central venous pressure** (CVP). If EDP (and thus EDV) is increased, the force of the next contraction and stroke volume also increases (Fig. 14.1b). This is known as the **Frank–Starling** relationship. The graph relating stroke volume to EDP is called a **Starling** or **ventricular function** curve. **Stroke work** (see Chapter 13) is often plotted instead of stroke volume as a useful indicator of function. The force of contraction is related to the degree of stretch of the muscle, and **Starling's Law of the**

Heart is quoted as 'The energy released during contraction depends on the initial fibre length'.

The length–tension relationship

In contrast to skeletal muscle, the relationship between cardiac muscle length and the generation of force can only partly be explained in terms of the **sliding filament theory** of muscle function. Briefly, this is based on the premise that as the muscle fibre is stretched, more crossbridges are able to form between myosin and actin (Fig. 14.1c), and thus force increases. Cardiac muscle, however, has a much steeper relationship between stretch and force production than skeletal muscle, and an additional mechanism must therefore be involved. This mechanism takes the form of an increase in Ca^{2+} sensitivity of cardiac muscle, and involves troponin C (see Chapter 11). Thus when the muscle fibre is stretched, a smaller increase in intracellular Ca^{2+} is required to generate the same amount of force (Fig. 14.1d). This mechanism seems to be of greater importance in the heart than that involving increased crossbridge formation, and provides a greater sensitivity to small degrees of stretch.

The importance of Starling's Law

The most important consequence of Starling's Law is that the stroke volumes of the left and right ventricles are matched. Small transient differences in output occur all the time, e.g. during breathing, or rising from a supine position when CVP falls. However, if right ventricular output was greater than that from the left for any significant period, pulmonary blood volume and pressure would rise dramatically, and fluid would be forced into the lung interstitium and alveoli (**pulmonary oedema**). This does not normally happen because any increase in pulmonary blood pressure increases the filling pressure, and hence EDV, of the left ventricle. Left ventricular stroke volume then increases according to Starling's Law. Over a couple of beats it continues to increase until it has matched right ventricular output, so preventing any further rise in pulmonary venous pressure, and equilibrium is regained.

For the same reasons a rise in CVP will cause an increase in stroke volume from both right and left ventricles, that is, an increase in cardiac output. Starling's Law will therefore also contribute to the rise in cardiac output during exercise when CVP may increase, and to the initial fall in cardiac output seen on standing, when CVP falls due to blood pooling in the legs. Starling's Law is an important compensatory mechanism in heart failure (see Chapter 44).

Effect of afterload

Another consequence of Starling's Law is that, within limits, stroke volume can be maintained in the face of an increase in blood pressure, or **afterload**. If blood pressure, or the resistance to outflow, increases, the left ventricle has to pump against a higher load, and the amount of blood ejected is reduced (i.e. the **ejection fraction**, the proportion of EDV actually pumped out, falls). There is therefore more blood left in the ventricle at the end of systole (**end-systolic volume**, ESV) than in the previous beat. This means that when the ventricle is filled again during diastole there is already more blood than usual in the ventricle, and this, combined with the consequent rise in filling pressure due to the temporarily mismatched outputs (see above), means that the EDV is greater than that for the previous beat. As a result stroke volume and work increase due to the increased stretch of the ventricular wall by Starling's Law. Over the course of a few beats stroke volume therefore returns to its original value, though at the cost of an increased EDP and EDV.

Influence of the autonomic nervous system

The autonomic nervous system provides an external mechanism for regulating cardiac output, and is central to the control of blood pressure (see Chapters 26, 27). Sympathetic stimulation or application of epinephrine causes an increase in heart rate and contractile force, and the ventricular function curve is shifted upwards (Fig. 14.1b). A change in the ability of cardiac muscle to generate force *without any change in length* is called a change in **contractility**. Agents that alter contractility are known as **inotropic agents** or **inotropes**. Positive inotropes increase contractility, and include the sympathetic neurotransmitter norepinephrine. Negative inotropes decrease force, and include an increase in acidity. Note that parasympathetic stimulation does not decrease ventricular contractility, as parasympathetic innervation is sparse. The effects of the autonomic nervous system on heart rate and contractility, and inotropic and chronotropic agents, are discussed in more detail in Chapters 10 and 11.

In summary, it can be seen that only the ventricular filling pressure and changes in heart rate and cardiac muscle contractility will affect SV. As the output of the right ventricle will also be maintained in the face of a rise in left ventricular filling pressure (i.e. RV afterload) by the effect of Starling's Law, it becomes clear that CVP and the autonomic nervous system are the prime determinants of cardiac output (Fig. 14.1e).

15 Electrical conduction system in the heart

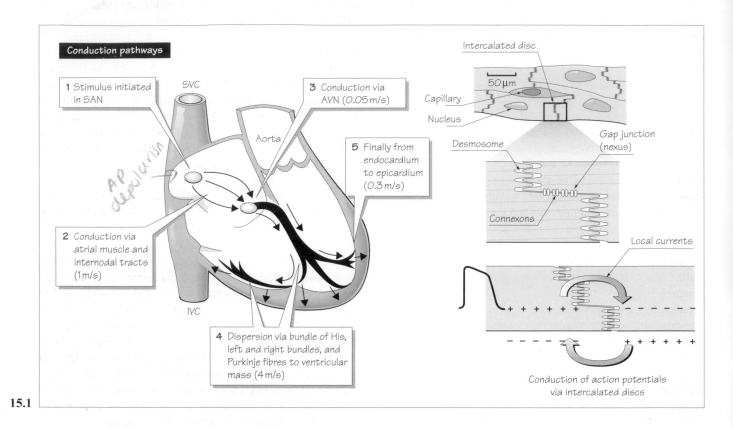

Conduction pathways

1 Stimulus initiated in SAN

SVC

3 Conduction via AVN (0.05 m/s)

Aorta

5 Finally from endocardium to epicardium (0.3 m/s)

2 Conduction via atrial muscle and internodal tracts (1 m/s)

IVC

4 Dispersion via bundle of His, left and right bundles, and Purkinje fibres to ventricular mass (4 m/s)

Intercalated disc

50 μm

Capillary

Nucleus

Desmosome

Gap junction (nexus)

Connexons

Local currents

+ + + + + + + +   − − − −

− − − − − −   + + + + + +

Conduction of action potentials via intercalated discs

15.1

Electrical conduction in cardiac muscle

Cardiac muscle cells are connected via **intercalated discs** (see Chapter 2). These incorporate regions where the membranes of adjacent cells are very close, called **gap junctions**. Gap junctions consist of proteins known as **connexons**, which form low-resistance junctions between cells. They allow the transfer of small ions and thus electrical current. As all cells are therefore electrically connected, cardiac muscle is said to be a **functional** (or electrical) **syncytium**. If an action potential (AP) is initiated in one cell, local currents via gap junctions will cause adjacent cells to depolarize, initiating their own AP. A wave of depolarization will therefore be conducted from cell to cell throughout the myocardium. The rate of conduction is partly dependent on gap junction resistance and the *size of the depolarizing current*. This is related to the **upstroke velocity of the AP** (phase 0). Drugs that slow phase 0 slow conduction (e.g. lignocaine, class I antiarrhythmics). Pathological conditions such as ischaemia may increase gap junction resistance, and slow or abolish conduction. Retrograde conduction does not normally occur because the original cell is refractory (see Chapter 10). Transfer of the pacemaker signal from the sinoatrial node and synchronous contraction of the ventricles is facilitated by **conduction pathways** formed from modified muscle cells.

Conduction pathways in the heart
Sinoatrial node

The heart beat is normally initiated in the **sinoatrial node** (SAN), which is located at the junction of the superior vena cava and the right atrium. The SAN is a group of muscle cells that extends for ~2 cm down the sulcus terminalis and is ~2 mm wide. The cells are small and elongated, and have fewer striations than normal cardiac muscle cells. The SAN has a rich capillary supply and sympathetic and parasympathetic (right vagal) nerve endings. The SAN generates an AP about once a second (see Chapter 10).

Atrial conduction

The impulse spreads from the SAN across the right and left atria at ~1 m/s. Conduction to the **atrioventricular node** (AVN) is facilitated by larger cells in the three **internodal tracts** of Bachman (anterior), Wenckebach (middle) and Thorel (posterior).

The atrioventricular node

The atria and ventricles are separated by a nonconducting band, the **annulus fibrosus**. The AVN marks the upper region of the only conducting route through this band. The AVN is similar in structure to the SAN, and is situated near the interatrial septum and the mouth of the coronary sinus. It is innervated by sympathetic and left vagal nerves. The complex arrangement of small cells and slow AP upstroke (see Chapter 10) result in a very slow conduction velocity (~0.05 m/s). This provides a functionally significant delay of ~0.1 s between contraction of the atria and ventricles, which is reflected by the **PR interval** of the **ECG**. Sympathetic stimulation increases conduction velocity and reduces the delay, whereas vagal stimulation slows conduction.

The bundle of His and Purkinje system

The bundle of His transfers the impulse from the AVN through the annulus fibrosus to the top of the interventricular septum. Close to the attachment of the septal cusp of the tricuspid valve it branches to form the **left and right bundle branches**. The left bundle divides further into the posterior and anterior fascicles. The bundles travel under the endocardium down the walls of the septum, and at the base divide into the multiple fibres of the **Purkinje system**. This distributes the impulse over the inner walls of the ventricles. Cells in the bundle of His and Purkinje system have a large diameter (~40 μm) and rapid AP upstroke velocity, and consequently a fast rate of conduction (~4 m/s). The impulse spreads from the Purkinje cells through the ventricular wall to the epicardium at 0.3–1 m/s, thereby initiating contraction.

Defects in conduction

Heart block

Complete **heart block (third degree)** occurs when conduction between atria and ventricles is abolished. This can result from ischaemic damage to nodal tissue or the bundle of His. In the absence of a signal from the SAN, the AVN and bundle of His can generate a heart rate of ~40 beats/min. Some Purkinje cells may also spontaneously generate APs, but at a rate of less than 20/min.

Abnormally slow conduction in the AVN can result in incomplete (**first-degree**) heart block, where the delay is much greater than normal, resulting in an extended PR interval of the ECG. **Second-degree** heart block occurs when only a fraction of the impulses from the atria are conducted, so that, for example, ventricular contraction is only initiated every second or third atrial contraction (**2 : 1 or 3 : 1 block**). **Wenckebach block** (Mobitz I) is another type of second-degree block, in which the PR interval progressively lengthens until there is no transmission from atria to ventricles and a QRS complex is missed; the cycle then begins again. Patients with first- or second-degree block are often asymptomatic (show no symptoms).

Bundle branch block. When one branch of the bundle of His does not conduct, the part of the ventricle that it serves will still be stimulated by conduction through the myocardium from unaffected areas. As this form of conduction is slower, activation is delayed and the QRS complex is broadened. This is called **left** or **right bundle branch block**.

Congenital accessory conduction pathways

AV nodal re-entrant tachycardia (AVNRT) and **Wolff–Parkinson–White (WPW)** or **pre-excitation syndrome** are **arrhythmias** (disturbances of the cardiac rhythm) resulting in periodic episodes during which the heart rate abruptly increases to 150–250 beats per minute. Individuals with AVNRT have an additional or **accessory conduction pathway** between the atrium and the AVN. The normal AV pathway (termed α) conducts rapidly and has a long refractory period, while the accessory (β) pathway conducts slowly and has a short refractory period. In these individuals, AVNRT can be initiated when a *premature impulse* (one generated too soon after the preceding impulse by mechanisms described in Chapter 46) is generated in the atrium. If the α pathway is still refractory from the preceding impulse, it will not conduct the premature impulse. This impulse may, however, travel slowly down the β pathway (which has recovered from the preceeding impulse), and then encounter the distal end of the α pathway. Sufficient time has now elapsed for this pathway to be no longer refractory, and the impulse is able to ascend the α pathway in a retrograde direction, allowing it to return to the atrium. From here it can continue to cycle through the α and β pathways. This recycling of an impulse is known as **re-entry** or a **circus movement**. The ventricles are excited with each circuit, causing the tachycardia (increased heart rate).

WPW syndrome is an analogous condition in which the AVN is normal, but there is a separate congenital accessory conduction pathway (the **bundle of Kent**) between an atrium and ventricle. This pathway is often situated on the left free wall of the heart. Impulses from the atrium are conducted to the ventricles via both the AVN and the bundle of Kent. The latter conducts more rapidly than the AVN so part of the ventricle is stimulated before the rest, resulting in a wide QRS complex (**pre-excitation**). A premature impulse can set up a circus movement in a similar fashion to AVNRT, but in WPW syndrome the re-entry circuit encompasses the AVN, His–Purkinje system, ventricles, bundle of Kent and atria.

Other arrhythmias

Many other arrhythmias are caused, promoted or potentiated by defects in the conduction system due to ischaemia or cell damage. The mechanisms, types and treatment of arrhythmias are discussed in Chapters 46 and 48.

16 The electrocardiogram

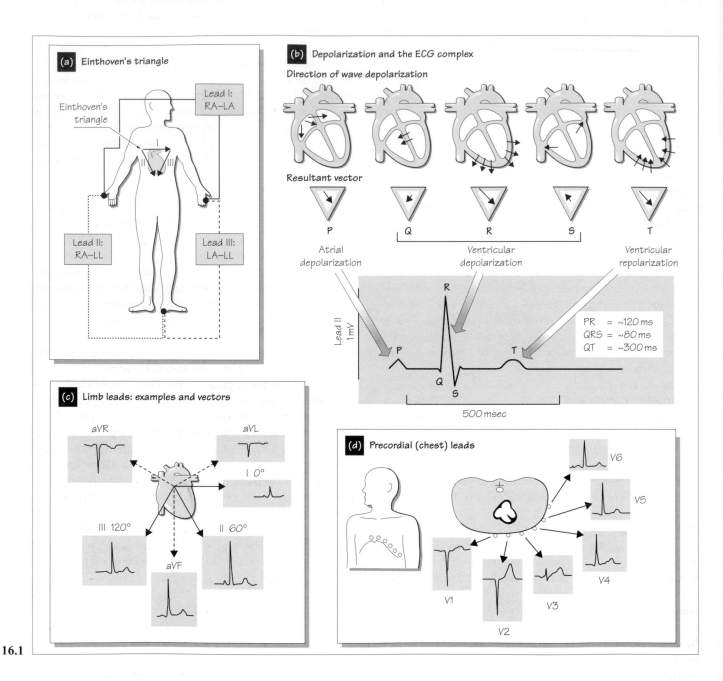

(a) Einthoven's triangle

Einthoven's triangle

Lead I: RA–LA

Lead II: RA–LL

Lead III: LA–LL

(b) Depolarization and the ECG complex

Direction of wave depolarization

Resultant vector

P   Q   R   S   T

Atrial depolarization

Ventricular depolarization

Ventricular repolarization

Lead II 1 mV

PR = ~120 ms
QRS = ~80 ms
QT = ~300 ms

500 msec

(c) Limb leads: examples and vectors

aVR   aVL

I 0°

III 120°   II 60°

aVF

(d) Precordial (chest) leads

V6

V5

V1   V4

V3

V2

16.1

The extracellular fluids contain salts, and therefore conduct electricity. As these fluids are distributed throughout the body, the body acts as a **volume conductor**. When cardiac muscle depolarizes, extracellular currents between depolarized and resting cells cause potentials that can be measured at the body surface. These form the basis of the **electrocardiogram** (ECG).

Recording the ECG

The ECG is based around the concept of an equilateral triangle

(**Einthoven's triangle**), with the heart as the current source at its centre (Fig. 16.1a). The points of the triangle are approximated by the limb leads, connected to the right arm, left arm and left leg. The potential difference between two leads will depend on the amplitude of the current, related to muscle mass, and the direction of current flow. There is a directional component because maximum potential occurs in line with the maximum current flowing between depolarized and resting tissue. The ECG thus has both amplitude and direction, and is a **vector quantity** (Fig. 16.1b).

By convention, the ECG is connected in such a way that a positive voltage causes an upward deflection, and the paper speed of the recorder is normally 25 or 50 mm/s. Note that the term **lead**, when used for the ECG, refers to a measurement made for a particular configuration, not to the wires connected to the patient.

The **classical bipolar leads** of the ECG approximate the potential difference across the sides of Einthoven's triangle, and are essentially looking at electrical activity in the heart from three different directions, separated by 60°. They are **Lead I**, measured as the potential difference between the right and left arm; **Lead II**, right arm and left leg; and **Lead III**, left leg and left arm. Lead II normally has the largest deflections, as it lies closest to the direction of ventricular depolarization. As the ventricles have the largest muscle mass, they give the largest current and thus voltage.

The **unipolar leads** use a single sensing electrode, and the voltage measured is the potential difference between this and an estimate of zero potential. Practically, the latter is obtained by connecting the limb leads together via a resistor. This approximates to the centre of the current source and hence Einthoven's triangle, i.e. the heart. Nine unipolar leads are commonly used clinically, consisting of six chest (**precordial**) leads, V1–V6, and the **augmented** leads **aVR**, **aVL**, and **aVF**. The chest leads use a separate sensing electrode placed on the chest (Fig. 16.1d), whereas the augmented leads use a limb lead as a sensing electrode (right arm, aVR; left arm, aVL; left leg, aVF), with the remaining two limb leads connected together to give the zero potential estimate. As the augmented leads measure between one point of Einthoven's triangle and the centre, they are seeing the heart at an angle rotated by 30° compared to the bipolar leads. The six limb leads together therefore give a view of the electrical activity of the heart every 30° (Fig. 16.1c).

General features of the ECG

The ECG trace has three main components that are related to the amplitude and direction of the wave of depolarization (vector) at that moment (Fig. 16.1b). The **P wave** is a small deflection due to depolarization of the atria. This is followed by the **QRS complex**, which is generally ~0.08 s in duration and reflects ventricular depolarization. It is the largest deflection because of the large ventricular muscle mass. The relative size of the Q, R and S components varies between leads, and is dependent on the orientation of the heart. In lead II the Q wave is seen as a small downward deflection, correlating to the left to right depolarization of the interventricular septum. The R wave is a strong upwards deflection, corresponding to depolarization of the main mass of the ventricles. The S wave is a small downward deflection in lead II, and relates to depolarization of the last part of the ventricles close to the base of the heart. The **T wave** corresponds to ventricular repolarization. Note that atrial repolariza-

tion is too diffuse to be seen. As the mass of the conducting system (sinoatrial and atrioventricular node, bundle of His) is very small, the associated currents are too small to cause any appreciable deflection in the ECG.

The **PR** and **ST segments** are normally **isoelectric**, i.e. at zero potential. There is no potential because no current is flowing; the relevant tissue (atria or ventricles) is either all depolarized or all at rest. The nonconducting *annulus fibrosus* prevents current flow between the atria and ventricles during the PR segment. The **PR interval** reflects the delay between atrial and ventricular depolarization, and is largely related to the delay in the atrioventricular node. It is measured from the beginning of the P wave to the beginning of the QRS complex, and ranges from 0.12 to 0.20 s. It shortens as heart rate increases.

The **ST segment** approximates to the plateau of the ventricular muscle action potential (AP), and is ~0.35 s. When the myocardium is injured, e.g. during ischaemia, some cells will be partially depolarized causing **injury currents** between them and undamaged tissue. This can either depress or elevate the ECG baseline. However, during the ST segment all cells are completely depolarized. This gives rise to an apparent elevation or depression of the ST segment, although it is actually the baseline that has altered. This is a common indication for acute myocardial damage such as a **myocardial infarction**.

Why the T wave is positive. The QRS complex in lead II is positive because the wave of depolarization progresses from the apex of the heart towards the base. As the T wave reflects repolarization it might be expected to be negative, because polarity is reversed. However, the length of the AP at the apex is longer than that at the base. Therefore although the apex depolarizes first, it repolarizes last, and the wave of repolarization progresses from the base towards the apex. The change in both polarity and direction cancel out, and the T wave is upwards. In pathological conditions where the AP is prolonged, or conduction from apex to base is slow, repolarization at the base may be delayed until after that at the apex. Under these conditions the T wave will be *inverted*.

The electrical axis of the heart

The angle of the ECG vector at its maximum amplitude is called the electrical axis of the heart. It corresponds to the point of maximum current developed during the heart beat, and hence depolarization of the main mass of the ventricles. It can be calculated from the three bipolar leads, which are at 60° to each other, and normally lies closest to lead II. Changes in the position of the heart will alter the axis, e.g. during breathing. An increase in mass of one of the ventricles will shift the axis in that direction. Thus left ventricular hypertrophy will cause **left axis deviation**, and right ventricular hypertrophy **right axis deviation**.

17 Haemodynamics

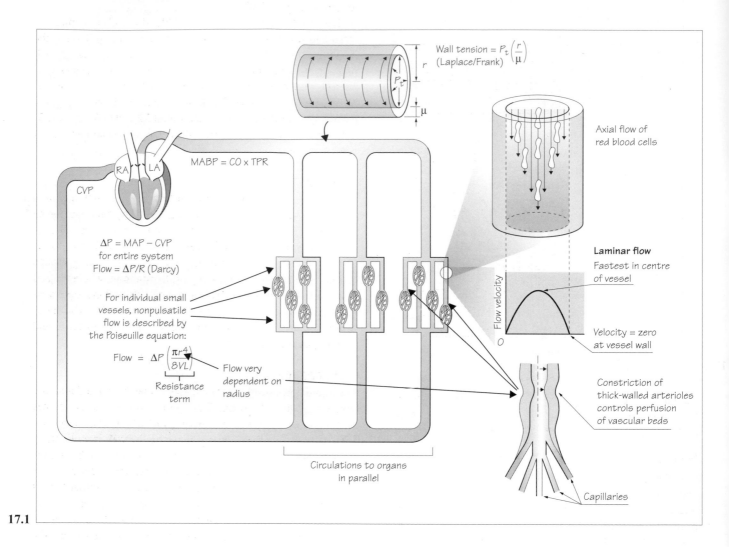

Wall tension $= P_t\left(\dfrac{r}{\mu}\right)$ (Laplace/Frank)

MABP = CO × TPR

$\Delta P = MAP - CVP$
for entire system
Flow $= \Delta P/R$ (Darcy)

For individual small vessels, nonpulsatile flow is described by the Poiseuille equation:

Flow $= \Delta P\left(\dfrac{\pi r^4}{8VL}\right)$

Resistance term

Flow very dependent on radius

Axial flow of red blood cells

Laminar flow
Fastest in centre of vessel

Flow velocity

Velocity = zero at vessel wall

Constriction of thick-walled arterioles controls perfusion of vascular beds

Circulations to organs in parallel

Capillaries

17.1

Relationships between pressure, resistance and flow

Haemodynamics is the study of the relationships between **pressure**, **resistance** and the **flow of blood** in the cardiovascular system. Although the properties of this flow are enormously complex, they can largely be derived from simpler physical laws governing the flow of liquids through single tubes.

When a fluid is pumped through a closed system, its flow (Q) is determined by the pressure head developed by the pump ($P_1 - P_2$ or ΔP), and by the resistance (R) to that flow, according to **Darcy's law** (analogous to Ohm's law):

$$Q = \Delta P/R$$

or for the cardiovascular system as a whole:

$$CO = (MABP - CVP)/TPR$$

where CO is cardiac output, $MABP$ is mean arterial blood pressure, TPR is total peripheral resistance and CVP is central venous pressure. Since CVP is ordinarily close to zero, $MABP$ is equal to $CO \times TPR$.

Resistance to flow is caused by frictional forces within the fluid, and depends on the viscosity of the fluid and the dimensions of the tube, as described by **Poiseuille's law**:

$$\text{resistance} = 8VL/\pi r^4$$

so that:

$$\text{flow} = \Delta P(\pi r^4/8VL)$$

Here, V is the viscosity of the fluid, L is the tube length, and r is the inner radius ($= 1/2$ the diameter) of the tube. Because flow depends on the 4th power of the tube radius in this equation, *small changes in radius have a powerful effect on flow*. For example, a 20% decrease in radius reduces flow by about 60%.

Considering the cardiovascular system as a whole, the different types or sizes of blood vessels (e.g. arteries, arterioles,

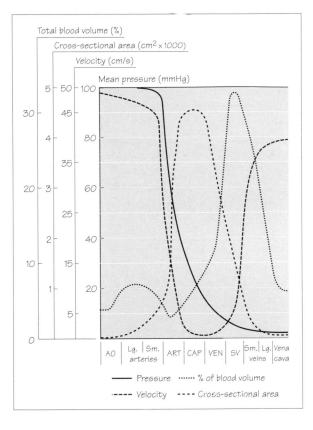

be accomplished, as a consequence of Poiseuille's law, by relatively small dilatations or constrictions of the arterioles within an organ or vascular bed.

Because there are so many small blood vessels (e.g. millions of arterioles, billions of venules, trillions of capillaries), the overall cross-sectional area of the vasculature reaches its peak in the microcirculation. As the velocity of the blood at any level in the system is equal to the total flow (the cardiac output) divided by the cross-sectional area at that level, the blood flow is slowest in the capillaries (see Fig. 17.2), favouring O_2/CO_2 exchange and tissue absorption of nutrients. The capillary transit time at rest is 0.5–2 s.

Blood viscosity

Very viscous fluids like motor oil flow more slowly than less viscous fluids like water. **Viscosity** is caused by frictional forces within a fluid which resist flow. Although the viscosity of plasma is similar to that of water, the viscosity of blood is normally three to four times that of water, because of the presence of blood cells, mainly erythrocytes. In **anaemia**, where the cell concentration (haematocrit) is low, viscosity and therefore vascular resistance decrease, and CO rises. Conversely, in the high-haematocrit condition **polycythaemia**, vascular resistance and blood pressure are increased.

Laminar flow

As liquid flows steadily through a long tube, frictional forces are exerted by the tube wall. These, in addition to viscous forces within the liquid, set up a *velocity gradient* across the tube (see Fig. 17.1) in which the fluid adjacent to the wall is motionless, and the flow velocity is greatest at the centre of the tube. This is termed **laminar flow**, and occurs in the microcirculation, except in the smallest capillaries. One consequence of laminar flow is that erythrocytes tend to move away from the vessel wall and align themselves edgewise in the flow stream. This reduces the effective viscosity of the blood in the microcirculation (the **Fåhraeus–Lindqvist effect**), helping to minimize resistance.

Wall tension

In addition to the pressure gradient along the length of blood vessels, there exists a pressure difference across the wall of a blood vessel. This *transmural pressure* is equal to the pressure inside the vessel minus the interstitial pressure. The transmural pressure exerts a circumferential *tension* on the wall of the blood vessel that tends to distend it, much as high pressure within a balloon stretches it. According to the **Laplace/Frank law**:

$$\text{wall tension} = P_t(r/\mu)$$

where P_t is the transmural pressure, r is the vessel radius, and μ is the wall thickness. In the aorta, where P_t and r are high, atherosclerosis may cause thinning of the arterial wall, and the development of a bulge or **aneurysm** (Chapter 34). This increases r and decreases μ, setting up a vicious cycle of increasing wall tension which, if not treated, may result in vessel rupture.

capillaries) are arranged sequentially, or in *series*. In this case, the resistance of the entire system is equal to the *sum of all the resistances* offered by each type of vessel:

$$R_{total} = R_{arteries} + R_{arterioles} + R_{capillaries} + R_{venules} + R_{veins}$$

Calculations taking into account the estimated lengths, radii and numbers of the various sizes of blood vessels show that the arterioles, and to a lesser extent the capillaries and venules, are primarily responsible for the resistance of the cardiovascular system to the flow of blood. In other words, $R_{arteriole}$ makes the largest contribution to R_{total}. Because according to Darcy's law the pressure drop in any section of the system is proportional to the resistance of that section, the steepest fall in pressure is in the arterioles (see Fig. 17.2).

Although the various sizes of blood vessel are arranged in series, each organ or region of the body is supplied by its own major arteries that emerge from the aorta. The vascular beds for the various organs are therefore arranged in *parallel* with each other. Similarly, the vascular beds within each organ are mainly arranged into parallel subdivisions (e.g. the arteriolar resistances $R_{arteriole}$ are in parallel with each other). For 'n' vascular beds arranged in parallel:

$$1/R_{total} = 1/R_1 + 1/R_2 + 1/R_3 + 1/R_4 \ldots 1/R_n$$

An important consequence of this relationship is that the bloodflow to a particular organ can be altered (by adjustments of the resistances of the arterioles in that organ) without greatly affecting pressures and flows in the rest of the system. This can

18 Blood pressure and flow in the arteries and arterioles

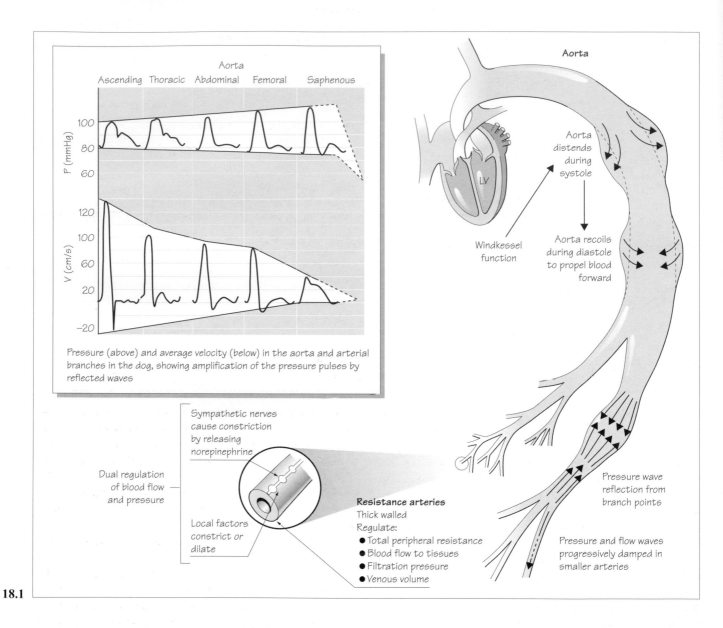

Pressure (above) and average velocity (below) in the aorta and arterial branches in the dog, showing amplification of the pressure pulses by reflected waves

Factors controlling arterial blood pressure

The mean arterial blood pressure is equal to the product of the cardiac output (about 5 L/min at rest) and the total peripheral resistance (TPR). Since the total drop of mean pressure across the systemic circulation is about 100 mmHg, TPR is calculated to be 100 mmHg/5000 ml/min, or 0.02 mmHg/ml/min. The unit mmHg/ml/min is referred to as a peripheral resistance unit (PRU), so that TPR is normally about 0.02 PRU.

Systolic pressure is mainly influenced by the stroke volume, the left ventricular ejection velocity, and aortic/arterial stiffness, and rises when any of these increase. Conversely, diastolic pressure rises with an increase in TPR. Arterial pressure falls progressively during diastole (see Fig. 13.1), so that a shortening

of the diastolic interval associated with a rise in the heart rate also increases diastolic pressure.

Blood pressure and flow in the arteries

The bloodflow in the aorta and the larger arteries is *pulsatile*, as a result of the rhythmic emptying of the left ventricle.

As blood is ejected from the left ventricle during systole, it hits the column of blood already present in the ascending aorta, creating a *pressure wave* in the aortic blood which is rapidly (at between 4 and 10 m/s) conducted towards the arterioles. As this pulse pressure wave passes each point along the aorta and the major arteries, it sets up a transient pressure gradient that briefly propels the blood at that point forward, causing a pulsatile *flow*

Table 18.1 Endogenous substances and other factors affecting arteriolar tone.

	Vasoconstrictors	Vasodilators

Neurotransmitters	Sympathetic
	  Norepinephrine
	ATP
	Neuropeptide Y
		Parasympathetic and sensory (limited distribution)
		  Acetylcholine (acts via NO)
		Substance P
		Calcitonin gene-related peptide
		Vasoactive intestinal peptide

Hormones	Epinephrine (most blood vessels) Angiotensin II Vasopressin (antidiuretic hormone)	Epinephrine (in skeletal muscle, coronary, hepatic arteries) Atrial natriuretic peptide
Endothelium-derived substances	Endothelin Endothelium-derived constricting factor (chemical identity unknown)	Endothelium-derived relaxing factor (NO) Prostaglandin I_2 (prostacyclin) Endothelium-derived hyperpolarizing factor (chemical identity unknown)
Metabolites and related factors	Hypoxia (pulmonary arteries only)	Hypoxia (other vessels) Adenosine, hyperosmolarity, H^+ ions, lactic acid, K^+ ions, CO_2
Other locally produced factors	Histamine (veins, pulmonary arteries) Prostaglandin $F_{2\alpha}$, thromboxane A_2 5-Hydroxytryptamine Growth factors (e.g. PDGF)	Histamine (arterioles) Prostaglandin E_2 Bradykinin
Other factors	Pressure (myogenic response) Moderate cold (skin)	Increased flow Heat (skin)

wave. The blood in the arteries therefore moves forward in short bursts, separated by longer periods of stasis, so that its average velocity in the aorta is about 0.2 m/s.

The pressure wave also causes the elastic arterial wall to bulge out, thereby storing some of the energy of the wave. The arterial wall then rebounds, releasing part of this energy to drive the blood forward during diastole (*diastolic runoff*). This pumping mechanism of the elastic arteries is termed the **Windkessel** function (Fig. 18.1).

The large arteries also absorb and dissipate some of the energy of the pressure wave. This progressively damps the oscillations in flow, as shown by the lower traces in the inset to Fig. 18.1. However, as the upper traces illustrate, the pulse pressure wave becomes somewhat *larger* as it moves down the aorta and major arteries (e.g. the saphenous artery), before it then progressively dies out along the smaller arteries. This occurs in part because a fraction of the pressure wave is *reflected* back towards the heart at arterial branch points. In the aorta and large arteries, the reflected wave *summates* with the forward-moving pulse pressure wave, increasing its amplitude. Once the blood has entered the smaller arteries, however, the damping properties of the arterial wall predominate, and progressively depress the oscillations in flow and pressure, so that these die out completely by the time the blood reaches the microcirculation.

Arterioles and vascular resistance

The mean blood pressure falls progressively along the arterial system. The decline is particularly steep in the smallest arteries and the arterioles (diameter < 100 μm), because these vessels present the greatest resistance to flow (see Fig. 17.2). The walls of the arterioles are very thick in relation to the diameter of the lumen, and these vessels can therefore constrict powerfully, dramatically increasing this resistance. Because the arterioles are normally partially constricted, their resistance can also be decreased by vasodilating stimuli.

The role of the arterioles in setting the vascular resistance has several important implications:

1 Constriction or dilatation of all, or a large proportion, of the arterioles in the body will affect the TPR and the blood pressure.
2 Constriction of the arterioles in one organ or region will selectively direct the flow of blood away from that region, while dilatation will have the opposite effect.
3 Changes in arteriolar resistance in a region affect the 'downstream' hydrostatic pressure within the capillary beds and veins in that region. Changes in the pressure within the capillaries affect the movement of fluid from the blood to the tissues (see Chapter 20). Because the veins are very compliant, their volume is very sensitive to alterations in pressure (see Chapter 21). Thus, arteriolar constriction in a region of the body will both promote the movement of fluid from its tissue spaces into its exchange vessels, and also decrease its venous volume. Both effects work to increase the blood supply to other parts of the body.

Table 18.1 lists important endogenous substances and factors which affect arteriolar tone.

19 The microcirculation and lymphatic system

(a) Structure of the microcirculation

- Smooth muscle cells
- Small arterioles
- Terminal arterioles
- Precapillary sphincter
- Metarteriole (present in some tissues)
- Capillaries
- Capillaries
- Lymphatic capillaries
- Postcapillary venules
- Venule

(b) Capillary structure

- Sinusoid or discontinuous capillary
- Fenestrated capillary
- Red blood cells
- Large lipophobic molecules
- Small lipophobic molecules
- Very slow diffusion: large lipophobic molecules
- Very fast diffusion: gases, lipophilic molecules
- Fused invaginations
- Slow diffusion small lipophobic molecules
- Basement membrane
- Intercellular cleft
- Glycocalyx
- Tight junction (especially tight in brain = blood–brain barrier)

Continuous capillary

19.1

The **microcirculation** comprises the **smallest arterioles**, and the **exchange vessels**, including the **capillaries** and the **postcapillary venules**. The transfer of gases, water, nutrients, waste materials and other substances between the blood and body tissues carried out by the exchange vessels is the ultimate function of the cardiovascular system.

Organization of the microcirculation

Blood enters the microcirculation via small arterioles, the walls of which contain smooth muscle cells. These vessels are densely innervated by the sympathetic system, particularly in the splanchnic and cutaneous vascular beds. Sympathetically mediated constriction of each small arteriole reduces the bloodflow to many capillaries.

In the vast majority of tissues, the smallest or **terminal** arterioles divide to give rise to sets of capillaries (Fig. 19.1a, left). The terminal arteriole itself acts as a functional precapillary sphincter for its entire cluster of capillaries. Terminal arterioles are not innervated, and their tone is controlled by local metabolic factors (see Chapter 22). Under basal conditions, terminal arterioles constrict and relax periodically. This **vasomotion** causes the flow of blood through the cluster of capillaries to fluctuate.

In a few tissues, however (e.g. mesentery), capillaries branch from **thoroughfare vessels** which run from small arterioles to venules (Fig. 19.1a, right). The proximal (arteriolar) end of such a vessel is termed a **metarteriole**, and it is wrapped intermittently in smooth muscle cells. The capillaries have a ring of smooth muscle called a **precapillary sphincter** at their origin, but thereafter lack smooth muscle cells. Constriction of the precapillary sphincter controls the flow of blood through that capillary.

The capillaries join to form *postcapillary venules*, which also lack smooth muscle cells. These merge to form *venules*, which contain smooth muscle cells and are sympathetically innervated.

Movement of solutes across the capillary wall

Water, gases and solutes (e.g. electrolytes, glucose, proteins) cross the walls of exchange vessels mainly by **diffusion**, a passive process by which substances move down their concentration gradients. O_2 and CO_2 can diffuse through the lipid bilayers of the endothelial cells. These and other **lipophilic** substances (e.g. general anaesthetics) therefore cross the capillary wall very rapidly. However, the lipid bilayer is impermeable to electrolytes and small **hydrophilic** (lipid-insoluble) molecules such as glucose, which therefore cross the walls of **continuous** capillaries (Fig. 19.1b, bottom) 1000–10 000 times more slowly than does O_2. Hydrophilic molecules cross the capillary wall mainly by diffusing between the endothelial cells. This process is slowed by *tight junctions* between the endothelial cells which impede diffusion through the intercellular clefts. Diffusion is also retarded by the **glycocalyx**, a dense network of fibrous macromolecules coating the luminal side of the endothelium. This tortuous diffusion pathway (the **small pore system**) acts as a sieve which admits molecules of molecular weight (MW) less than 10 000.

Even large proteins (e.g. albumin, MW 69 000) can cross the capillary wall, albeit very slowly. This suggests that the capillary wall also contains a small number of **large pores**, although these have never been directly visualized. It has been proposed that large pores exist transiently when membrane invaginations on either side of the endothelial cell fuse, temporarily creating a channel through which large molecules diffuse.

The endothelial cells of **fenestrated** capillaries (found in kidneys, intestines and joints) contain pores called **fenestrae** (Fig. 19.1b, upper right). Fenestrated capillaries are about 10 times more permeable than are continuous capillaries to small hydrophilic molecules, because these can move through the fenestrae. **Sinusoidal** or **discontinuous** capillaries (liver, bone marrow, spleen) are very highly permeable, because they have wide spaces between adjacent endothelial cells through which proteins and even erythrocytes can pass (Fig. 19.1b, upper left).

The blood–brain barrier

The composition of the extracellular fluid in the brain must be kept extremely constant in order to allow stable neuronal function. This is made possible by the existence of the **blood–brain barrier** (BBB), which tightly controls the movement of ions and solutes across the walls of the continuous capillaries within the brain and the choroid plexus. The BBB has two important features. First, the junctions between the endothelial cells of cerebral capillaries are extremely tight (resembling the *zonae occludens* of epithelia), preventing any significant movement of hydrophilic solutes. Second, specialized membrane transporters exist in cerebral endothelial cells which allow the controlled movement of inorganic ions, glucose, amino acids and other substances across the capillary wall. Thus, the relatively uncontrolled diffusion of solutes present in other vascular beds is replaced in the brain by a number of specific transport processes. This can present a therapeutic problem, as most drugs are excluded from the brain (e.g. many antibiotics).

The BBB is interrupted in the **circumventricular organs**, areas of the brain which need to be influenced by blood-borne factors, or to release substances into the blood. These include the *pituitary* and *pineal* glands, the *median eminence*, the *area postrema*, and the *choroid plexus*. The BBB can break down with large elevations of blood pressure, osmolarity or P_{CO_2}, and in infected areas of the brain.

The lymphatic system

Approximately 8 L of fluid containing solutes and plasma proteins is filtered from the microcirculation into the tissue spaces each day. This returns to the blood via the **lymphatic system**. Most body tissues contain *lymphatic capillaries* (Fig. 19.1a). These are blind-ended bulbous tubes 15–75 µm in diameter, with walls formed of a monolayer of endothelial cells. Interstitial fluid, plasma proteins and bacteria can easily enter the lymphatic capillaries via the gaps between these cells, the arrangement of which then prevents these substances from escaping. These vessels merge to form *collecting lymphatics*, the walls of which contain smooth muscle cells and one-way valves (as do the larger lymphatic vessels). The sections between these valves constrict strongly, forcing the lymph towards the blood. Lymph is also propelled by compression of the vessels by muscular contraction, body movement, and tissue compression. Lymph then enters the larger *afferent lymphatics*, which flow into the **lymph nodes**. Here, foreign particles and bacteria are scavenged by phagocytes, and can initiate the production of activated lymphocytes. These enter the lymph fluid for transport into the circulation, where they mount an immune response.

Much of the lymph fluid is returned to the blood via capillary absorption in the lymph nodes. The remaining fluid enters *efferent lymphatics*, most of which eventually merge into the *thoracic duct*. This duct empties into the left subclavian vein in the neck. Lymphatics from parts of the thorax, the right arm, and the right sides of the head and neck merge forming the *right lymph duct*, which enters the right subclavian vein. The lymphatic system is also important in the absorption of lipids from the intestines. The *lacteal* lymphatics are responsible for transporting about 60% of digested fat into the venous blood.

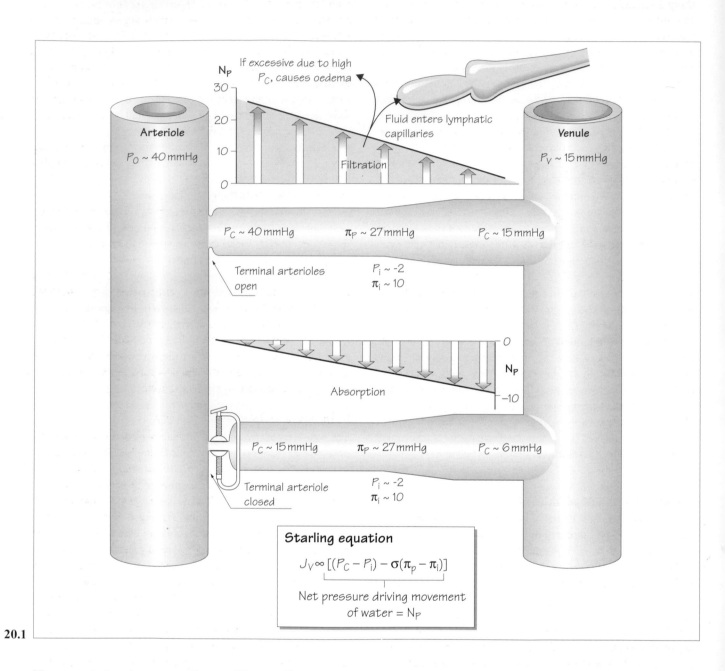

Starling equation

$$J_V \propto [(P_C - P_i) - \sigma(\pi_p - \pi_i)]$$

Net pressure driving movement of water = N_P

Movement of water across the capillary wall

The capillary wall (here taken to include also the wall of post-capillary venules) is very permeable to water molecules, which are able to pass easily in both directions through the plasma membranes of the endothelial cells. However, although individual water molecules can move freely between the plasma and the tissue spaces, the *net* flow of water across the capillary wall is quite small. This flow is determined by a balance between two forces or pressures which are exerted across the wall of the capillaries. These are a **hydrostatic pressure**, which tends to drive water out of the capillary, and a colloid **osmotic pressure**, which

tends to draw water in from the surrounding tissue spaces. The sum of these two pressures at each point along the capillary is equal to a net pressure that will be directed either out of or into the capillary. The net flow of water is then proportional to this net pressure. The relationship between net flow (J_v) and the hydrostatic and osmotic pressures is described by the **Starling equation**:

$$J_v \propto [(P_c - P_i) - \sigma (\pi_p - \pi_i)]$$

The **hydrostatic force** ($P_c - P_i$) is equal to the difference between the blood pressure inside the capillary (P_c) and the pressure in the interstitium around the capillary (P_i). When capillaries are open (upper part of Fig. 20.1), P_c ranges from about 35 mmHg at the arteriolar end of the capillaries to about 15 mmHg in the venules. P_i is slightly subatmospheric in many tissues (−5–0 mm Hg), due to a suction of fluid from the interstitium by the lymphatic capillaries. The greater pressure inside the capillary tends to drive water out into the tissues.

As described in Chapter 19, the capillary wall acts as a *semipermeable membrane* or barrier to free diffusion, across which electrolytes and small molecules pass with much greater ease than plasma proteins. A substance dissolved on one side of a semipermeable membrane exerts an osmotic pressure that draws water across the membrane from the other side. This osmotic pressure is proportional to the concentration of the substance in solution, and is also a function of its permeability. Substances that can easily permeate a barrier (in this case the capillary wall) exert little osmotic pressure across it, whereas those which permeate less readily exert a larger osmotic pressure. For this reason, the osmotic force across the capillary wall is largely a result of the relatively impermeant plasma proteins, in particular albumin. The osmotic pressure exerted by plasma proteins is referred to as the **oncotic** or **colloid osmotic** pressure.

The osmotic force across the capillary wall is equal to the difference between the oncotic pressure of the plasma (π_p) and that of the interstitium (π_i), multiplied by a factor, the **reflection coefficient** (σ), which is a measure of how difficult it for the proteins to cross the capillary wall. Substances that cannot cross the membrane at all have a reflection coefficient of 1, while those that pass freely have a reflection coefficient of zero. σ ranges from 0.8–0.95 for most plasma proteins, while ($\pi_p - \pi_i$) is typically about 13 mmHg.

Water filtration and absorption

Until recently, it was thought that the balance of forces described by the Starling equation was such that fluid tended to be *filtered* (i.e. to move out of the capillary) at the arteriolar end of the capillaries, and to be *absorbed* (move into the capillaries) at the venular end. However, the osmotic pressure term in the Starling equation is now thought to be somewhat smaller than previously estimated. Therefore, in most tissues, capillaries and venules that are being perfused with blood will be mainly filtering plasma (Fig. 20.1, upper part). On the other hand, certain sites such as the kidneys or the intestinal mucosa are specialized for water reabsorption. Here the osmotic pressure term is large, because plasma proteins are continually being washed out of the interstitium, so that net reabsorption occurs.

It is also the case that the balance between filtration and reabsorption is a dynamic one, mainly because the hydrostatic pressure within the capillaries is variable. Arteriolar vasodilatation, which increases intracapillary hydrostatic pressure, increases filtration, while arteriolar vasoconstriction favours absorption.

For example, arterioles often demonstrate *vasomotion* (i.e. random opening and closing). During periods of arteriolar *constriction*, capillary pressure *falls*, favouring the *absorption* of interstitial fluid. The lower part of Fig. 20.1 illustrates this principle, showing that arteriolar constriction sufficient to reduce capillary hydrostatic pressure to the values shown would result in absorption of fluid, especially at the venous end of the capillary. This absorption tends to be transient, however, because as fluid moves into the capillaries P_i falls and π_i increases. Both effects progressively diminish absorption.

Assumption of the upright posture increases the transcapillary hydrostatic pressure gradient in the lower extremities, thereby immediately increasing filtration in these regions. However, this effect is partially compensated for by a rapid constriction of the arterioles of the leg, which is mediated by a local sympathetic axon reflex. This reduces bloodflow and attenuates the rise in capillary hydrostatic pressure in these areas.

By the same token, fluid tends to accumulate in the tissue spaces of the upper body and face during the night, since assumption of the supine position increases capillary hydrostatic pressures above the heart. This causes morning 'puffiness'.

Normally, there is a slight predominance of filtration over absorption in the body as a whole. Of about 4000 L of plasma entering the capillaries daily as the blood recirculates, a *net* filtration of 8 L occurs. This fluid is returned to the vascular compartment through the lymphatic system.

Pulmonary and systemic oedema

The hydrostatic and osmotic pressures in the capillaries of the pulmonary circulation are atypical. Both P_c (~7 mmHg) and P_i (~8 mmHg) are low, while π_i is high (~18 mmHg), because these vessels are highly permeable to plasma proteins. The balance of forces slightly favours filtration. In **congestive heart failure**, the output of both the left and right ventricles is markedly reduced (see Chapter 44). Failure of the left ventricle results in an increase in left ventricular end-diastolic pressure. This pressure backs up into the lungs, causing increased pulmonary venular and capillary pressures. This promotes filtration in these vessels, causing an accumulation of fluid in the lungs (**pulmonary oedema**) which dramatically worsens the dyspnoea (breathlessness) and inadequate tissue oxygenation characteristic of congestive heart failure. Similarly, failure of the right ventricle increases systemic venous and therefore capillary pressure, leading to systemic oedema, particularly of the lower extremities.

Oedema of the legs is also caused by **varicose veins**, a condition in which the venous valves are unable to operate properly because the veins become swollen and overstretched. By interfering with the effectiveness of the skeletal muscle pump, the incompetence of the valves leads to increases in venous and capillary hydrostatic pressure, resulting in the rapid development of oedema during standing.

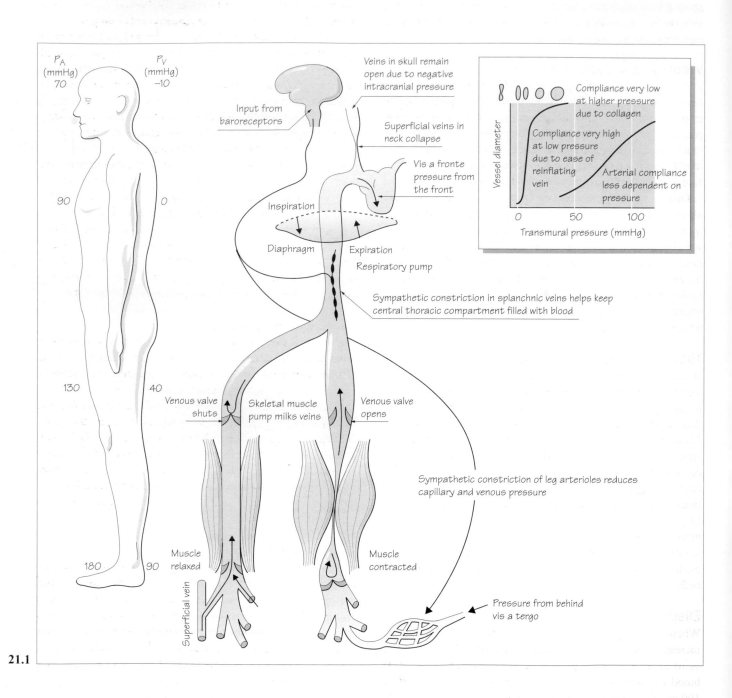

21.1

The venules and veins return the blood from the microcirculation to the right atrium. They do not, however, serve merely as passive conduits. Instead, they have a crucial active role in stabilizing and regulating the **venous return** of blood to the heart.

The venous system differs from the arterial system in two important respects. First, the total volume (and cross-sectional area) of the venous system is much greater than that of the arterial system. This is because there are many more venules than arterioles; venules also tend to have larger internal diameters than arterioles. Second, the veins are quite thin walled, and can therefore expand greatly to hold more blood if their internal pressure rises.

As a result of its large cross-sectional area, the venous system offers much less resistance to flow compared to the arterial system. The pressure gradient required to drive the blood through the venous system (15 mmHg) is therefore much smaller than the pressure needed in the arterial system (80 mmHg). The average pressure in the venae cavae at the level of the heart (the central venous pressure) is usually close to 0 mmHg (i.e. atmospheric pressure). The flow of blood back to the heart is aided by the presence of one-way **venous valves** in the arms and especially the legs, which prevent backflow.

Venous arterial compliance

The graph in Fig. 21.1 (upper right) illustrates the relationship between pressure and volume in a typical vein and artery. The slope of the volume/pressure curve is referred to as the **compliance**. Compliance is a measure of **expandability**. Veins are much more compliant than arteries at low pressures (0–10 mmHg). Small increases in venous pressure in this range therefore cause large increases in venous blood volume.

One reason for high venous compliance is that their thin walls allow veins to collapse at low internal pressures. Only small increases in pressure are needed to 'reinflate' a collapsed vein with blood until it has nearly rounded up. At higher pressures, however, venous compliance decreases dramatically (see graph) because the slack in rigid collagen fibres in the venous wall is rapidly taken up. This limit on the expandability of the veins is important in limiting the pooling of blood in the veins of the legs which occurs during standing.

The veins as capacitance vessels

Because of their large volumes and high compliance, the veins/venules accommodate a much larger volume of the blood (~70% of the total) than do the arteries/arterioles (~12%). They are therefore termed **capacitance vessels**, and are able to serve as *blood volume reservoirs*. During exercise, and in hypotensive states (e.g. during haemorrhage), sympathetically mediated constriction of the veins/venules, notably in the *splanchnic* (including the gastrointestinal tract and liver) and *cutaneous* circulations, displaces blood into the rest of the cardiovascular system. In particular, the resulting reduction of the venous volume increases the volume of blood in the *central thoracic compartment* (i.e. the heart and pulmonary circulation), thereby boosting cardiac output, assisting perfusion of other essential vascular beds, and helping to maintain the blood pressure.

Effects of posture

When the upright position is assumed, the pull of gravity increases the absolute pressures within *both* the arteries and veins of the lower extremities. The average arterial and venous blood pressures in a normal adult standing quietly are about 100 and 0 mmHg at the level of the heart, while in the feet the pressures are about 190 and 90 mmHg, respectively. However, gravity does not affect the *pressure gradient* driving the blood circulation, because the *difference* between the arterial and venous pressures is similar (100 mmHg) at both levels. Standing therefore does not stop blood from flowing back to the heart.

The increased pressure within the veins of the lower extremities causes them to distend, so that about 500 ml of blood is shifted into this part of the circulation. The rise in hydrostatic pressure within the capillaries of the lower extremities increases

fluid filtration, causing a progressive loss of plasma volume into the tissues of the legs and feet. The resulting loss of fluid from the central thoracic compartment lowers cardiac output.

These potentially harmful effects are limited by the baroreceptor and cardiopulmonary reflexes, which respond to a fall in the pulse pressure (see Chapter 26). These cause an *increased heart rate* and widespread *vasoconstriction*. This limits the loss of blood from the central thoracic compartment and slightly raises MAP and TPR. The cardiac output falls by about 20%. A local *sympathetic axon reflex* also reduces bloodflow to the lower extremities, limiting fluid filtration.

In the upright position, the reduction of intravascular pressures above the heart causes the partial collapse of superficial veins, although the deeper veins remain partly open because their walls are anchored to surrounding tissues. Standing also causes a downward displacement into the spinal canal of the cerebrospinal fluid bathing the CNS, creating a negative pressure inside the rigid cranium that prevents cerebral veins from collapsing. Because cerebral venous pressure is not able to fall as much as arterial pressure, cerebral bloodflow decreases by 10–20%.

The skeletal muscle pump

Even during quiet standing, the leg muscles are stimulated by reflexes to contract and relax rhythmically, causing swaying. During contraction, veins within the muscles are squeezed, forcing blood towards the heart, as the venous valves prevent retrograde flow. Upon relaxation, these veins expand, drawing in blood from venules and from superficial veins that communicate with the muscle veins via collaterals (Fig. 21.1). This *skeletal muscle pump* thus 'milks' the veins, driving blood towards the heart to assist venous return. The skeletal muscle pump is greatly potentiated during walking and running, dramatically lowering the venous pressure in the foot to levels as low as 30 mmHg.

The respiratory pump

During inspiration, downward displacement of the diaphragm causes the intrathoracic pressure to fall and the intra-abdominal pressure to rise. This increases the pressure gradient favouring venous return, and vena caval flow rises. An opposite effect occurs during expiration. During straining movements in which there is forced expiration against a closed glottis (e.g. the Valsalva manoeuvre), the rise in intrathoracic pressure severely reduces venous return.

Effect of cardiac contraction

Downward displacement of the ventricles during systole pulls on the atria, expanding them and drawing in blood from the venae cavae and pulmonary veins. When the valves between the atria and ventricles then open during diastole, the blood is drawn in from these veins by the expansion of the ventricles, further aiding venous return. Venous return is therefore driven not only by the upstream pressure, but also (to a smaller extent) by downstream suction.

22 Local control of bloodflow

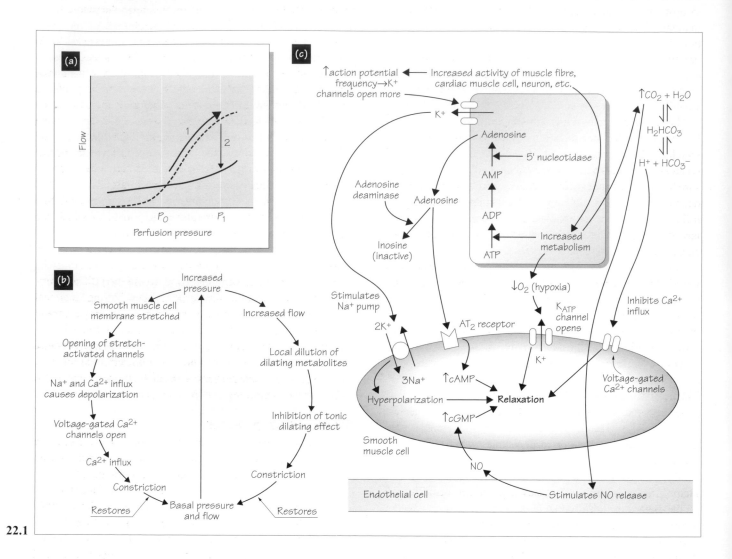

22.1

The activity of the sympathetic nervous system provides for centrally coordinated control of vascular tone (see Chapters 26, 27) and serves to maintain constant arterial blood pressure. There are, however, additional mechanisms that regulate vascular tone. Local mechanisms arise either from within the blood vessel itself, or from the surrounding tissue. These **local** mechanisms function primarily to regulate **flow**. Regulation tends to be most important in organs which require a constant blood supply, or in which metabolic needs may increase markedly (brain, kidneys, heart, skeletal muscles).

Local mechanisms have two main functions. First, under *basal conditions* they regulate local vascular resistance to maintain the bloodflow in many types of vascular beds at a nearly constant level over a large range of arterial pressures (50–170 mmHg). This tendency to maintain a *constant flow* during variations in pressure is termed **autoregulation**. Autoregulation prevents

major fluctuations in capillary pressure that would lead to uncontrolled movement of fluid into the tissues.

Second, when a tissue requires more blood to meet its metabolic needs, local mechanisms cause dilatation of resistance vessels and upregulate bloodflow. This response is referred to as **metabolic vasodilatation**. Autoregulation may persist under these conditions, but is adjusted to maintain flow around the new set point.

Autoregulation

Figure 22.1(a) illustrates the phenomenon of autoregulation. When the upstream pressure driving blood through a resistance artery is suddenly increased to P_1 from its starting level P_0, the artery dilates passively and bloodflow immediately rises as predicted by Poiseuille's law (arrow 1). Within a minute, however, the resistance artery responds to the increased pressure by *actively constricting* (arrow 2), thereby bringing bloodflow back down towards its initial level (solid line). Similarly, decreases in upstream pressure cause rapid compensatory dilatations to maintain flow. Autoregulation ensures that under basal conditions bloodflow remains nearly constant over a wide range of pressures, and is particularly important in the heart, the brain, and the kidneys. Two homeostatic negative feedback mechanisms are involved, the **myogenic response** and the effect of **vasodilating metabolites** (Fig. 22.1b).

The myogenic response is thought to be controlled mainly by sensors in the plasma membrane of smooth muscle cells, which react to changes in pressure and/or stretch. These include **stretch-activated channels**, which respond to increased pressure by opening to allow Na^+ and Ca^{2+} influx. The resulting cell depolarization opens voltage-gated Ca^{2+} channels, causing Ca^{2+} influx and vasoconstriction. The opposite process (i.e. hyperpolarization, closing of Ca^{2+} channels) occurs when pressure falls, causing vasodilatation.

Cellular metabolism results in the production of **vasodilating metabolites** or **factors** (Fig. 22.1c) which diffuse into the tissue spaces and affect neighbouring arterioles. If bloodflow increases, these substances tend to be washed out of the tissue, leading to an inhibition of vasodilatation that counteracts the rise in bloodflow. Conversely, decreased bloodflow causes a local accumulation of metabolites, leading to a homeostatic vasodilatation.

Metabolic and reactive hyperaemia

When metabolism in cardiac and skeletal muscle increases during exercise, tissue concentrations of vasodilating metabolites rise markedly. Similarly, focal changes in brain metabolism accompany diverse types of mental activity, causing enhanced local production of metabolites. The increased presence of such factors in the interstitium causes a powerful vasodilatation, termed **metabolic** or **functional hyperaemia**, allowing the rises in bloodflow necessary to supply the increased metabolic demand.

An accumulation of vasodilating metabolites also occurs during flow occlusion (e.g. caused by thrombosis). Release of occlusion then results in **reactive hyperaemia**; this is a large increase in bloodflow that hastens the re-establishment of cellular energy stores. This response is transient, persisting until levels of these metabolites fall back to normal levels.

Metabolic factors

Many factors contribute to metabolic vasodilatation. The most important factors are thought to be **adenosine**, **K^+ ions** and **hypercapnia** (increased P_{CO_2}). Local **hypoxia** (reduced P_{O_2})

can also relax vascular smooth muscle cells, partly by opening ATP-sensitive K^+ channels. **Inorganic phosphate, hyperosmolarity** and **lactic acid** may also act as metabolic vaso-dilators (not shown), although this is less well established.

Adenosine is a potent vasodilator that is released from the heart, skeletal muscles and brain during increased metabolism and hypoxia. It is thought to contribute to metabolic control of bloodflow in these organs. Adenosine is produced when AMP, which accumulates as a result of increased ATP breakdown, is dephosphorylated by the cell membrane enzyme **5′-nucleotidase**. It passes into the extracellular space, dilating neighbouring arterioles before being broken down to inosine by **adenosine deaminase**. It causes vasodilatation by acting on **A_2 receptors** to increase cAMP levels in vascular myocytes. Adenosine also has other actions in the body (e.g. inhibiting conduction in the atrioventricular node), some of which are mediated by **A_1 receptors** (which lower cAMP).

Ischaemia or increased activation of muscles and nerves causes K^+ ions to move out of cells. Resulting increases in the extracellular K^+ concentration (up to $10–15$ mM) dilate arterioles, partly by stimulating the Na^+,K^+-ATPase, during functional hyperaemia in skeletal muscle and brain tissue. **Hypercapnia** associated with **acidosis** occurs in brain tissue during stimulation of local metabolism, and also during **cerebral ischaemia** (stroke). These are thought to provide a powerful vasodilating stimulus, both by releasing **nitric oxide** from endothelial cells, and by directly inhibiting Ca^{2+} influx into arteriolar cells.

Other local mechanisms

There are also a number of mechanisms acting locally in selected vascular beds under specific circumstances. For example, during the inflammatory reaction, local infection or trauma causes the release of various **autocoids** (local hormones), including the arteriolar dilators **histamine, prostaglandin E_2, bradykinin** and **platelet activating factor**. These increase local bloodflow and increase postcapillary venular permeability, thereby increasing the access of leucocytes and antibodies to damaged and infected tissues. The generation of **bradykinin** by sweat glands during sweating promotes cutaneous vasodilatation. **Prostaglandin I_2** (PGI_2, prostacyclin) is synthesized and released in the renal cortex under conditions where renal bloodflow is reduced by vasoconstrictors. Prostacyclin has a vasodilating action that helps to maintain renal bloodflow. Conversely, the release of **serotonin** (5-hydroxytryptamine) and **thromboxane A_2** from platelets during haemostasis causes vasospasm, which helps to reduce bleeding (see Chapter 7).

23 Regulation of the vasculature by the endothelium

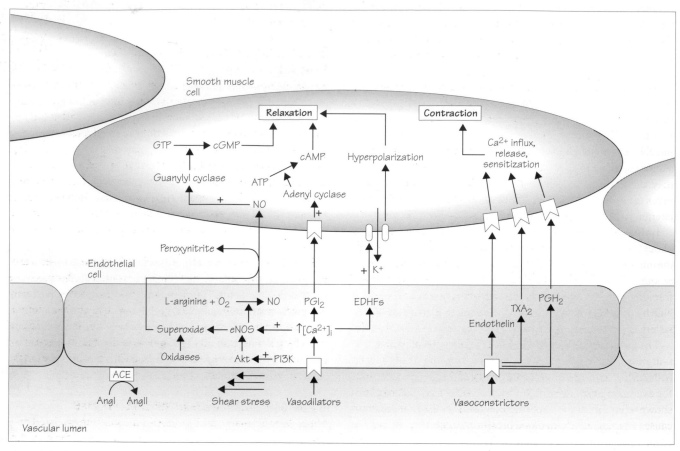

23.1

The inner surface of blood vessels is lined by a monolayer of endothelial cells and these are crucial in regulating vascular tone. When stimulated by substances present in the blood, or by the shear stress associated with the flow of blood, endothelial cells can release both constricting and dilating substances (Fig. 23.1). Important endothelial vasodilators include **endothelium-derived relaxing factor** (EDRF, now known to be **nitric oxide** or a closely related nitroso-containing compound), **prosta-cyclin** (PGI$_2$), and **endothelium-derived hyperpolarizing factor** (EDHF). The major endothelial vasoconstrictors are **endothelin-1, thromboxane A$_2$** (TXA$_2$), and **prostaglandin H$_2$**.

Endothelial cells also play a crucial role in suppressing platelet aggregation and thereby regulating haemostasis (see Chapter 7), and, as the major constituents of the capillary wall, control vascular permeability to many substances (Chapter 19).

Nitric oxide

Nitric oxide (chemical formula NO) is the most important vasodilator released by endothelial cells. NO is synthesized from the amino acid L-arginine and molecular oxygen by nitric oxide synthase (NOS). The most important form of NOS in the cardiovascular system is **endothelial NOS** (eNOS). This enzyme is responsible for a continual production and release of NO by endothelial cells (also by platelets and the heart). eNOS can be activated by a variety of substances that act on their receptors to increase the endothelial cell intracellular Ca^{2+} [Ca^{2+}]$_i$, leading to raised levels of the Ca^{2+}–calmodulin complex which stimulates the enzyme. The rise in [Ca^{2+}]$_i$ is initiated by Ca^{2+} release from the endoplasmic reticulum, and is subsequently sustained at a lower but still above basal level by Ca^{2+} influx via store-operated Ca^{2+} channels (see Chapter 12). Substances which cause vasodilatation in this way include locally released factors such as bradykinin, adenine, adenosine nucleotides, histamine, serotonin and the neurotransmitter substance P. Acetylcholine has a similar effect, although it is not known whether this has any physiological importance.

Shear forces exerted on the endothelium by the flow of blood also activate eNOS, and this is thought to make an important contribution to both basal NO release and local regulation of bloodflow. This effect is not caused by a rise in [Ca^{2+}]$_i$, but by cellular pathways activated by shear force-induced deformation of the endothelial cell cytoskeleton. One such pathway involves the sequential activation of the enzymes **phosphatidylinositol 3-kinase (PI3K)** and **Akt**, the latter of which stimulates eNOS via phosphorylation.

Once released from the endothelium, NO diffuses through the vascular wall and into the smooth muscle cells, where it activates the cytosolic enzyme **guanylyl cyclase**. This increases levels of cellular cyclic GMP, which causes relaxation by mechanisms described in Chapter 12.

NO is a free radical (i.e. it contains an unpaired electron), and is therefore very reactive. In particular, upon its release NO reacts very rapidly with **superoxide**, another free radical which is continually being produced by a variety of enzymes (including eNOS). This results in the formation of **peroxynitrite**, a substance which does not cause vasodilatation, and which in excess may damage cells. Any given molecule of NO therefore survives for only a few seconds, meaning that the effects of NO are exerted locally, and depend upon its continued production.

Inducible NOS (iNOS) is expressed in macrophages, lymphocytes, vascular smooth muscle and many other types of cells during inflammation. iNOS is capable of producing much greater amounts of NO, and probably contributes to the destruction of foreign organisms by the immune system. An overproduction of NO by iNOS in septic shock is thought to contribute to the severe hypotension characterizing this condition.

The formation of NO can be competitively antagonized by L-arginine analogues such as L-nitro arginine methyl ester (L-NAME); these have proved to be useful experimental tools for evaluating the roles of NO *in vitro* and *in vivo*. It has been shown, for example, that infusion of L-NAME in humans causes a sustained rise in blood pressure, suggesting that a tonic basal release of NO is acting to reduce the total peripheral resistance.

Pharmacological sources of NO

Organic nitrates such as **glyceryl trinitrate** and **isosorbide dinitrate** are acted on by the enzyme glutathione *S*-transferase in vascular smooth muscle to release nitrite ion (NO_2^-), which is then converted to NO to cause dilatation. These drugs, which dilate veins more effectively than arteries, are used to treat angina pectoris (see Chapter 39). The drug **sodium nitroprusside** releases NO spontaneously in both arterial and venous smooth muscle cells, and its powerful dilator effect on both arteries and veins is useful in the treatment of hypertensive emergencies and acute heart failure.

Other endothelium-derived relaxing factors

Prostacyclin is released from the endothelium by many of the factors that cause NO release. It promotes vasodilatation by increasing smooth muscle cell cyclic AMP levels, but its most important role is in limiting platelet attachment and aggregation. The endothelium also releases **endothelium-derived hyperpolarizing factor (EDHF)**, which opens K^+ channels on vascular smooth muscle cells. This causes these cells to hyperpolarize, resulting in relaxation (see Chapter 12). EDHF probably represents a diverse family of substances rather than a single molecule, and likely EDHFs include arachidonic acid metabolites, hydrogen peroxide and K^+ ions. EDHF is thought to be particularly important in causing dilatation of arterioles, where its influence may exceed that of NO.

Endothelium-derived constricting factors

Endothelin-1 is a peptide of 21 amino acids which is released by the endothelium in the presence of many vasoconstrictors, including angiotensin, vasopressin, thrombin and epinephrine. Endothelin is a potent vasoconstricting agent, particularly in veins and arterioles, and stimulates two subtypes of receptor on vascular smooth muscle cells, designated ET_A and ET_B. Endothelin causes vasoconstriction via G-protein-linked mechanisms similar to those activated by norepinephrine. The infusion of endothelin receptor antagonists into humans causes a sustained fall in total peripheral resistance, implying that ongoing endothelin release contributes to maintaining the blood pressure.

Endothelial cells are also capable of releasing other vasoconstricting substances, including **prostanoids** (thromboxane A_2 and prostaglandin H_2), and superoxide anions which may enhance constriction by breaking down NO. In addition, **angiotensin-converting enzyme** (ACE) present on the surface of endothelial cells converts is responsible for the production of the vasoconstrictor angiotensin II (see Chapter 28), as well the breakdown of the potent vasodilator bradykinin.

The endothelium in cardiovascular disease

Many diseases that disturb vascular function are associated with abnormalities of the endothelium. Dysfunction of the endothelium is thought to contribute to the early stages of **atherosclerosis**, while damage to the endothelium is a crucial factor leading to thrombus formation in the advanced atherosclerotic lesion (see Chapter 34). Plasma from patients with **diabetes mellitus** contains abnormally high levels of biochemical markers indicative of endothelial damage, and there is evidence, both in animal models of insulin-dependent diabetes and in patients with this disorder, that endothelium-dependent relaxation is blunted. This deficit in endothelial function is thought to contribute to the increased risks of atherosclerosis, neuropathy and hypertension that are associated with diabetes. The mechanisms leading to diabetes-associated endothelial dysfunction remain incompletely defined, but may include damage by raised levels of glucose and/or oxidized low density lipoproteins.

Endothelial dysfunction may also be important in causing **pre-eclampsia**, a disorder of pregnancy characterized by hypertension and increased blood clotting, which is the leading cause of maternal mortality. The endothelium is thought to play an important role in causing the fall in maternal blood pressure that normally occurs during pregnancy. This protective function may, however, be disrupted in patients suffering from pre-eclampsia, possibly due to the release of substances from the placenta which damage the endothelial cells.

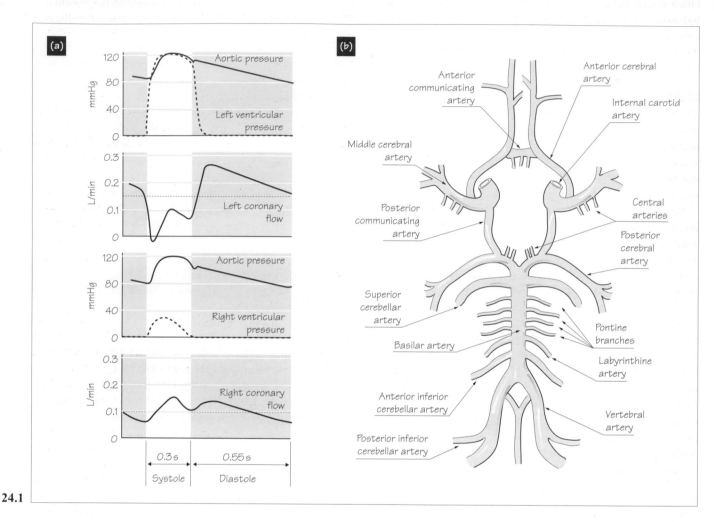

24.1

The vascular beds supplying the different organs of the body are structurally and functionally specialized, allowing an optimal matching of bloodflow with their individual requirements.

Coronary circulation

The **left** and **right coronary** arteries branch from the aorta just above the aortic valve. The left coronary artery gives rise to **left circumflex** and **anterior descending** branches which supply mainly the left ventricle and septum. The right coronary artery supplies mainly the right ventricle. Venous drainage of the heart occurs mainly (95%) into the right atrium via the **coronary sinus** and **anterior cardiac vein**. A small amount of venous blood also enters all cardiac chambers through **thebesian** and **anterior coronary** veins.

The *high capillary density* of the myocardium (~1 capillary per muscle cell), allows it to extract an unusually large fraction (about 70%) of the oxygen from its blood supply. The resting bloodflow to the heart is relatively high, and moreover increases approximately fivefold during strenuous exercise.

Figure 24.1(a) shows left and right coronary bloodflow during the cardiac cycle at a resting heart rate of 70 beats/min. During systole, the branches of the left coronary artery which penetrate the myocardial wall to supply the subendocardium of the left ventricle are strongly compressed by the high pressure within the ventricle and its wall. Left coronary bloodflow is therefore almost abolished during systole, so that 85% of flow occurs during diastole. Conversely, right coronary arterial flow rate is highest during systole, because the aortic pressure driving flow increases more during systole (from 80 to 120 mmHg) than the right ventricular pressure which opposes flow (from 0 to 25 mmHg).

With a heart rate of 70 beats/min, systole and diastole last 0.3 and 0.55 s, respectively. As the heart rate increases during exercise or excitement, however, the duration of diastole shortens more than that of systole. At 200 beats/min, for example, systole and diastole both last for 0.15 s. In order to cope with the greatly increased oxygen demand of the heart, which occurs simultaneously with a marked reduction in the time available for left coronary perfusion, the coronary arteries/arterioles dilate dramatically to allow for a pronounced rise in bloodflow. Dilatation is caused by *vasodilating factors*, including **adenosine**, **hypoxia** and **K+**, which are generated as a result of *increased cardiac metabolism*. *The heart therefore regulates its own blood supply via a well-developed* **metabolic hyperaemia** (see Chapter 22).

Skeletal muscle circulation

The skeletal muscles comprise about 50% of body weight, and at rest receive 15–20% of cardiac output. At rest, skeletal muscle arterioles have a high basal tone as a result of tonic sympathetic vasoconstriction. At any one time, most muscle capillaries are not perfused, due to intermittent constriction of precapillary sphincters (vasomotion).

Because the muscles form such a large tissue mass, their arterioles make a major contribution to total peripheral resistance. Sympathetically mediated alterations in their arteriolar tone therefore play a crucial role in regulating total peripheral resistance and blood pressure during operation of the baroreceptor reflex. The muscles thus serve as a '*pressure valve*' that can be closed to increase blood pressure and opened to lower it.

With *rhythmic exercise*, compression of blood vessels during the contraction phase causes the bloodflow to become intermittent. However, increased muscle metabolism causes the generation of *vasodilating factors*; these factors cause an enormous increase in bloodflow during the relaxation phase, especially to the white or *phasic* fibres involved in movement. With maximal exercise, the skeletal muscles receive 80–90% of cardiac output. Vasodilating factors include **K+ ions**, **CO$_2$** and **hyperosmolarity**. In working muscle their effects completely *override* sympathetic vasoconstriction, while arterioles in nonworking muscle remain sympathetically constricted so that their bloodflow does not increase.

Sustained compression of blood vessels during *static* (isometric) muscle contractions causes an occlusion of flow that rapidly results in muscle fatigue.

Cutaneous circulation

Apart from supplying the relatively modest metabolic requirements of the skin, the main function of the cutaneous vasculature is to maintain a constant body temperature. **Thermoregulation** is aided by the presence of **arteriovenous anastomoses** (AVAs). AVAs are coiled, thick-walled thoroughfare blood vessels, which connect arterioles and veins directly, bypassing the capillaries. AVAs are located mainly in the skin of the *hands*, *feet*, *lips*, *nose* and *ears*. When open, AVAs allow a high-volume bloodflow into a cutaneous venous *plexus* (network) from which heat can be radiated to the environment.

The sympathetic nervous system acts through α_1-*receptors* to control the resistance of AVAs and also cutaneous arterioles and veins. A fall in temperature, sensed by peripheral and hypothalamic thermoreceptors, causes a hypothalamically mediated increase in sympathetic outflow to the skin. This causes the AVAs and cutaneous arterioles and veins to constrict. This minimizes the loss of body heat by producing a pronounced decrease in cutaneous bloodflow, which can fall to one-tenth of its thermoneutral level of 10–20 ml/min/100 g.

With an increased temperature, decreased sympathetic outflow allows the AVAs and other cutaneous blood vessels to open, bringing blood to the skin to increase sweating and heat loss. High temperatures also activate **cholinergic sympathetic fibres** to these areas of the skin. These stimulate sweating, leading to the local formation of **bradykinin**, which further promotes vasodilatation. The flow of blood to the skin can increase up to 30-fold with increases in temperature.

Local skin temperature also directly affects cutaneous blood vessels, which dilate to heat and constrict as temperature falls. Prolonged cold, however, causes a paradoxical vasodilatation. Cutaneous vessels are also constricted by the baroreceptor reflex, helping to increase TPR and shift blood to the vital organs during haemorrhage or shock.

Cerebral circulation

The brain receives about 15% of cardiac output. The **basilar** and **internal carotid arteries** entering the cranium join to form an arterial ring, the **circle of Willis**, from which arise the **anterior**, **middle** and **posterior cerebral arteries** that supply the cranium (Fig. 24.1b). This arrangement helps to defend the cerebral blood supply, which if occluded causes immediate unconsciousness and irreversible tissue damage within minutes.

The brain, especially the neuronal grey matter, has a very high capillary density (~3000–4000 capillaries/mm^3), and *arteriolar autoregulation* is highly developed, allowing cerebral bloodflow to be maintained constant at arterial pressures between about 50 and 170 mmHg. Autoregulation is both myogenic and metabolic; the **K+** and **CO$_2$** concentrations in the surrounding brain are particularly important in causing functional hyperaemia (see Chapter 22). The effect of CO$_2$ is in part caused by NO release from endothelial cells. Hyperventilation, which reduces arterial CO$_2$, can cause a marked cerebral vasoconstriction and temporary unconsciousness. Sympathetic regulation of the bloodflow to the brain is probably of minor importance.

The brain and spinal cord float in the **cerebrospinal fluid** (CSF), which is contained within the rigid cranium and the spinal canal. Because the cranium is rigid and its contents are incompressible, the volume of blood within the brain remains roughly constant, and increases in arterial inflow are compensated for by decreases in venous volume. By increasing the tissue mass, brain tumours increase the intracerebral pressure and reduce cerebral bloodflow. Increased intracerebral pressure is partially compensated for by the **Cushing reflex**, a characteristic rise in arterial pressure associated with a reflex bradycardia.

25 The pulmonary and fetal circulations

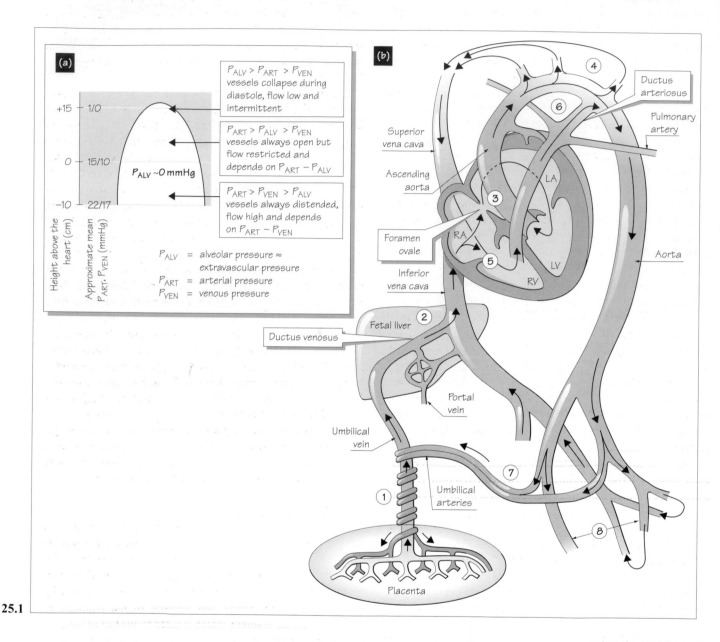

(a)

$P_{ALV} > P_{ART} > P_{VEN}$
vessels collapse during diastole, flow low and intermittent

$P_{ART} > P_{ALV} > P_{VEN}$
vessels always open but flow restricted and depends on $P_{ART} - P_{ALV}$

$P_{ART} > P_{VEN} > P_{ALV}$
vessels always distended, flow high and depends on $P_{ART} - P_{VEN}$

$P_{ALV} \sim 0 \, mmHg$

P_{ALV} = alveolar pressure ≈ extravascular pressure
P_{ART} = arterial pressure
P_{VEN} = venous pressure

Height above the heart (cm)
Approximate mean P_{ART}, P_{VEN} (mmHg)

+15 — 1/0
0 — 15/10
−10 — 22/17

(b)

Ductus arteriosus
Pulmonary artery
Superior vena cava
Ascending aorta
LA
Foramen ovale
RA
Aorta
LV
RV
Inferior vena cava
Fetal liver
Ductus venosus
Portal vein
Umbilical vein
Umbilical arteries
Placenta

25.1

The lungs contain two circulations. The **bronchial circulation** arises from the aorta, comprises about 1% of cardiac output, and supplies the metabolic needs of the airways. It drains partly into the superior vena cava through bronchial veins, and partly into pulmonary veins. The **pulmonary circulation** receives the entire output of the right ventricle. Its high density capillary network surrounds the lung alveoli, allowing the O_2-poor blood from the pulmonary arteries to exchange CO_2 for O_2. The pulmonary veins return highly oxygenated blood to the left atrium. The pulmonary circulation contains about 800 ml of blood in recumbent subjects, falling to about 450 ml during quiet standing.

The pulmonary circulation

Mean pulmonary arterial pressure is ~15 mmHg, and left atrial pressure is ~5 mmHg. The right ventricle is able to drive its entire output through the pulmonary circulation utilizing a pressure head of only 10 mmHg, because the resistance of the pulmonary circulation is only 10–15% that of the systemic circulation. This arises because the vessels of the pulmonary microcirculation are short and relatively wide bore, with little resting tone. They are also very numerous, so that their total cross-section is similar to that of the systemic circulation. The walls of both arteries and veins are thin and distensible, and contain comparatively little smooth muscle.

The low pressure within the pulmonary circulation means that regional perfusion of the lungs in the upright position is greatly affected by gravity (Fig. 25.1a). The extravascular pressure throughout the lungs is similar to the alveolar pressure (~0 mmHg). However, the intravascular pressure is low in the lung apices, which are above the heart, and high in the lung bases, which are below the heart. Pulmonary vessels in the lung apices therefore collapse during diastole, causing intermittent flow. Conversely, vessels in the bases of the lungs are perfused throughout the cardiac cycle, and are distended. A small increase in pulmonary arterial pressure during exercise is sufficient to open up apical capillaries, allowing more O_2 uptake by the blood.

The low hydrostatic pressure in pulmonary capillaries (mean of 7–10 mmHg) does not lead to net fluid reabsorption, because it is balanced by a low extravascular hydrostatic pressure and an unusually high interstitial plasma protein oncotic pressure (~18 mmHg). The lung capillaries therefore produce a small net flow of lymph, which is drained by an extensive pulmonary lymphatic network. During left ventricular failure or mitral stenosis, however, the increased left atrial pressure backs up into the pulmonary circulation, increasing fluid filtration and leading to **pulmonary oedema**.

Neither the sympathetic nervous system nor myogenic/metabolic autoregulation play a role in regulating pulmonary vascular resistance or flow. The pulmonary vasculature is, however, well supplied with sympathetic nerves. When stimulated, these decrease the compliance of the vessels, limiting the pulmonary blood volume so that more blood is available to the systemic circulation.

The most important mechanism regulating pulmonary vascular tone is **hypoxic pulmonary vasoconstriction** (HPV), a process by which pulmonary vessels *constrict* in response to alveolar **hypoxia**. This unique mechanism (*systemic* vessels typically *dilate* to hypoxia) diverts blood away from poorly ventilated regions of the lungs, thereby maximizing the **ventilation–perfusion ratio**. HPV is probably caused by the release of an unidentified endothelium-derived constricting factor. Hypoxia-mediated inhibition of smooth muscle K+-channel activity, resulting in membrane depolarization, may also be involved.

The fetal circulation

A diagram of the fetal circulation is shown in Fig. 25.1(b). The fetus receives O_2 and nutrients from, and discharges CO_2 and metabolic waste products into, the maternal circulation. This exchange occurs in the **placenta**, a thick spongy pancake-shaped structure lying between the fetus and the uterine wall. The placenta is composed of a space containing maternal blood, which is packed with **fetal villi**, branching tree-like structures containing fetal arteries, capillaries and veins. They receive the fetal blood from branches of the two **umbilical arteries**, and drain back into the fetus via the **umbilical vein**. Gas and nutrient exchange occurs between the fetal capillaries in the villi and the maternal blood surrounding and bathing the villi.

The fetal circulation differs from that of adults in that *the right and left ventricles pump the blood in parallel rather than in series*. This arrangement allows the heart and head to receive more highly oxygenated blood, and is made possible by three structural *shunts* unique to the fetus, the **ductus venosus**, the **foramen ovale**, and the **ductus arteriosus** (highlighted in Fig. 25.1b).

Blood leaving the placenta (**1**) via the umbilical vein is 80% saturated with O_2. About half of this flows into the fetus' liver. The rest is diverted into the inferior vena cava via the **ductus venosus** (**2**), mixing with poorly oxygenated venous blood returning from the fetus' lower body. When the resulting relatively oxygen-rich mixture (about 67% saturated) enters the right atrium, most of it does not pass into the right ventricle as it would in the adult, but is directed into the left atrium via the **foramen ovale**, an opening between the fetal atria (**3**). Blood then flows into the left ventricle, and is pumped into the ascending aorta, from which it perfuses the head, the coronary circulation, and the arms (**4**). Venous blood from these areas re-enters the heart via the superior vena cava. This blood, now about 35% saturated with O_2, mixes with the fraction of blood from the inferior vena cava not entering the foramen ovale (**5**), and flows into the right ventricle, which pumps it into the pulmonary artery. Instead of then entering the lungs, as it would in the adult, about 90% of the blood leaving the right ventricle is diverted into the descending aorta through the **ductus arteriosus** (**6**). This occurs because pressure in the pulmonary circulation is higher than that in the systemic circulation, as a result of pulmonary vasoconstriction and the collapsed state of the lungs. About 60% of blood entering the descending aorta then flows back to the placenta for oxygenation (**7**). The rest, now 58% saturated with O_2, supplies the fetus' trunk and legs (**8**).

Circulatory changes at birth

Two events at birth quickly cause the fetal circulation to assume a quasi-adult pattern. First, the pulmonary vascular pressure falls well below the systemic pressure because of the initiation of breathing and the resulting pulmonary vasodilatation. Together with constriction of the ductus arteriosus caused by increased blood O_2 levels, this reversal of the pulmonary–systemic pressure gradient, which is aided by the loss of the low-resistance placental circulation, abolishes the bloodflow from the pulmonary artery into the aorta within 30 min after delivery.

Second, tying off the umbilical cord stops venous return from the placenta, abruptly lowering inferior vena caval pressure. Together with the fall in pulmonary resistance, this lowers right atrial pressure, causing within hours functional closure of the foramen ovale. The ductus venosus also closes with the abolition of venous return from the placenta.

Although these fetal circulatory shunts are *functionally* closed soon after birth, complete *structural* closure only occurs after several months. In 20% of adults, the structural closure of the foramen ovale remains incomplete, although this is of no haemodynamic consequence.

26 Cardiovascular reflexes

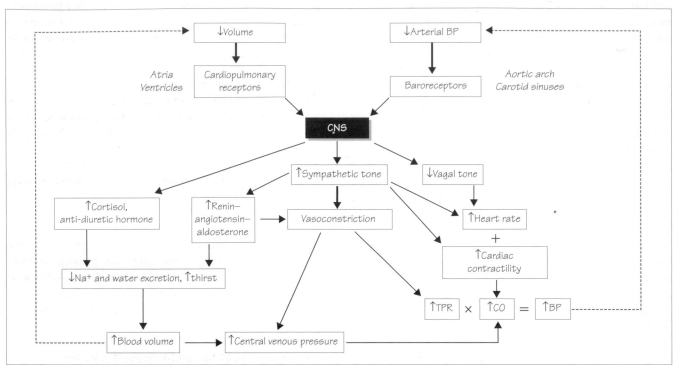

26.1

The cardiovascular system is centrally regulated by **autonomic reflexes**. These work with local mechanisms (see Chapter 22) to minimize fluctuations in the mean arterial blood pressure (MABP) and volume, and to maintain adequate cerebral and coronary perfusion. **Intrinsic** reflexes, including the **baroreceptor**, **cardiopulmonary** and **chemoreceptor** reflexes, respond to stimuli originating from within the cardiovascular system. Less important **extrinsic** reflexes mediate the cardiovascular response to stimuli originating elsewhere (e.g. pain, temperature changes). Figure 26.1 illustrates the responses of the baroreceptor and cardiopulmonary reflexes to a reduction in blood pressure and volume, as would occur, for example, during haemorrhage.

Cardiovascular reflexes involve three components:
1 afferent nerves (termed 'receptors') sense a change in the state of the system, and communicate this to the brain, which
2 processes this information and implements an appropriate response, by
3 altering the activity of efferent nerves controlling cardiac, vascular and renal function, thereby causing homeostatic responses which reverse the change in state.

Intrinsic cardiovascular reflexes

The baroreceptor reflex
This reflex acts rapidly to minimize moment-to-moment fluctuations in the MABP. **Baroreceptors** are afferent (sensory) nerve endings in the walls of the **carotid sinuses** (thin-walled dilatations at the origins of the internal carotid arteries) and the **aortic arch**. These **mechanoreceptors** sense alterations in wall stretch caused by pressure changes, and respond by modifying the frequency at which they fire action potentials. Pressure elevations increase impulse frequency; pressure decreases have the opposite effect.

When MABP decreases, the fall in baroreceptor impulse frequency causes the brain to reduce the firing of vagal efferents supplying the sinoatrial node, thus causing tachycardia. Simultaneously, the activity of sympathetic nerves innervating the heart and most blood vessels is increased, causing increased cardiac contractility and constriction of both arteries and veins. Stimulation of renal sympathetic nerves increases renin release, and consequently angiotensin II production and aldosterone secretion (see Chapter 28). The resulting tachycardia, vasoconstriction and fluid retention act together to raise MABP. Opposite effects occur when arterial blood pressure rises. The baroreceptors quickly show partial *adaptation* to new pressure levels. Therefore alterations in frequency are greatest while pressure is changing, and tend to moderate when a new steady-state pressure level is established. If unable to prevent MABP from changing to a new level, the reflex will within several hours become *reset* to maintain pressure around this level. It therefore plays little part in long-term regulation of MABP.

There are two types of baroreceptors. *A fibres* have large, myelinated axons and are activated over lower levels of pressure. *C fibres* have small, unmyelinated axons and respond over higher levels of pressure. Together, these provide an input to the brain, which is most sensitive to pressure changes between 80 and 150 mmHg. The brain is able to reset the baroreflex to allow increases in MABP to occur, e.g. during exercise and the defence reaction. Ageing, hypertension and atherosclerosis decrease arterial wall compliance, reducing baroreceptor reflex sensitivity.

Cardiopulmonary reflexes

Diverse intrinsic cardiovascular reflexes originate in the heart and lungs. Cutting the vagal afferent fibres that mediate these **cardiopulmonary reflexes** causes an increased heart rate and vasoconstriction, especially in skeletal muscle, renal and mesenteric vascular beds. The *net* effect of the cardiopulmonary reflexes is therefore thought to be a **tonic depression** of the *heart rate* and *vascular tone*. The receptors for these reflexes are located mainly (but not entirely) in *low-pressure regions* of the cardiovascular system, and are well placed to sense the *blood volume* in the central thoracic compartment. These reflexes are thought to be particularly important in controlling blood volume and vascular tone, and act together with the baroreceptors to stabilize the blood pressure. However, these reflexes have been studied mainly in animals, and their specific individual roles in humans are incompletely understood.

Specific components of the cardiopulmonary reflexes include:
1 Atrial mechanoreceptors with nonmyelinated vagal afferents, which respond to increased atrial volume/pressure by causing bradycardia and vasodilatation.
2 Mechanoreceptors in the left ventricle and coronary arteries with mainly nonmyelinated vagal afferents, which respond to increased ventricular diastolic pressure and afterload by causing a vasodilatation.
3 Ventricular chemoreceptors which are stimulated by substances such as bradykinin and prostaglandins released during cardiac ischaemia. These receptors activate the **coronary chemoreflex**. This response, also called the **Bezold–Jarisch effect**, occurs after the IV injection of many drugs, and involves marked bradycardia and widespread vasodilatation.
4 Pulmonary mechanoreceptors, which when activated by marked lung inflation, especially if oedema is present, cause tachycardia and vasodilatation.
5 Mechanoreceptors with myelinated vagal afferents, located mainly at the juncture of the atria and great veins, which respond to increased atrial volume and pressure by causing a sympathetically mediated tachycardia (the **Bainbridge reflex**). This reflex also helps to control blood volume; its activation decreases the secretion of **antidiuretic hormone** (vasopressin), **cortisol** and **renin**, causing a diuresis. Although this reflex is powerful in dogs, it has been difficult to demonstrate its effects in humans.

Chemoreceptor reflexes

Chemoreceptors activated by **hypoxia**, **hypocapnia** and **acidosis** are located in the aortic and carotid bodies. These receptors are stimulated during asphyxia, hypoxia and severe hypoten-sion. The resulting **chemoreceptor reflex** is mainly involved in stimulating breathing, but also has cardiovascular effects. These include sympathetic constriction of (mainly skeletal muscle) arterioles, splanchnic venoconstriction and a tachycardia resulting indirectly from the increased lung inflation. This reflex is important because its effects help maintain the bloodflow to the brain at arterial pressures too low to activate the baroreceptors.

The CNS ischaemic response

A powerful generalized peripheral vasoconstriction is stimulated by brainstem hypoxia. This response develops during severe hypotension, helping to maintain the flow of blood to the brain during shock. It also causes the **Cushing reflex**, in which vasoconstriction and hypertension develop when increased cerebrospinal fluid pressure (e.g. due to a brain tumour) produces brainstem hypoxia.

Extrinsic reflexes

Stimuli that are external to the cardiovascular system also exert effects on the heart and vasculature via extrinsic reflexes. Moderate pain causes tachycardia and increases MABP; however, severe pain has the opposite effects. Cold causes cutaneous and coronary vasoconstriction, possibly precipitating angina in susceptible individuals.

Central regulation of cardiovascular reflexes

The view that the brainstem contains a specific **vasomotor centre** responsible for controlling cardiovascular aspects of autonomic function is obsolete. It is now known that cardiovascular autonomic control arises as a result of interactions between areas of the brainstem, the hypothalamus, the cerebral cortex and the cerebellum.

The afferent nerves carrying impulses from cardiovascular receptors terminate in the **nucleus tractus solitarius** (NTS) of the medulla. Neurons from the NTS project to areas of the brainstem which control both parasympathetic and sympathetic outflow, influencing their level of activation. The **nucleus ambiguus** and **dorsal motor nucleus** contain the cell bodies of the preganglionic vagal parasympathetic neurons, which slow the heart when the cardiovascular receptors report an increased blood pressure to the NTS. Neurons from the NTS also project to areas of **ventrolateral medulla**; from these descend bulbo-spinal fibres which influence the firing of the sympathetic preganglionic neurons in the intermediolateral (IML) columns of the spinal cord.

These neural circuits are capable of mediating the basic cardiovascular reflexes. However, the NTS, the other brainstem centres and the IML neurons receive descending inputs from the hypothalamus, which in turn is influenced by impulses from the limbic system of the cerebral cortex. Input from these higher centres modifies the activity of the brainstem centres, allowing the generation of integrated responses in which the functions of the cardiovascular system and other organs are coordinated in such a way that the appropriate responses to changing conditions can be orchestrated.

27 Autonomic control of the cardiovascular system

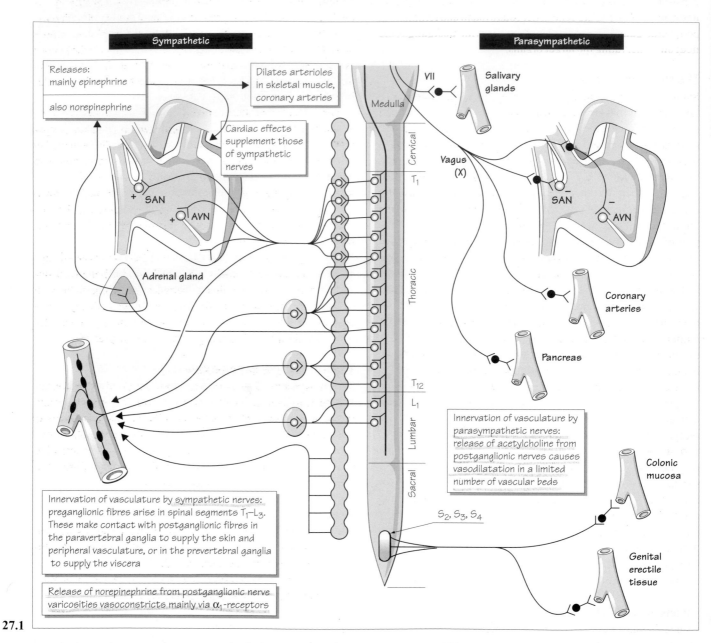

27.1

The **autonomic nervous system** (ANS) comprises a *system of efferent nerves* that regulate the involuntary functioning of most organs, including the heart and vasculature. The cardiovascular effects of the ANS are deployed for two purposes.

First, the ANS provides the effector arm of the cardiovascular *reflexes*, which responds mainly to activation of receptors in the cardiovascular system (see Chapter 26). They are designed to maintain an *appropriate blood pressure*, and play a crucial role in homeostatic adjustments to *postural changes* (see Chapter 21), *haemorrhage* (see Chapter 30) and *changes in blood gases*. The

autonomic circulation is able to override local vascular control mechanisms in order to serve the needs of the body as a whole.

Second, ANS function is also regulated by signals initiated within the brain as it reacts to *environmental stimuli* or *emotional stress*. The brain can selectively modify or override the cardiovascular reflexes, producing specific patterns of cardiovascular adjustments, which are sometimes coupled with behavioural responses. Complex responses of this type are involved in *exercise* (see Chapter 29), *thermoregulation* (see Chapter 24), the '*fight or flight*' *(defence) response*, and '*playing dead*'.

The ANS is divided into **sympathetic** and **parasympathetic** branches. The nervous pathways of both branches of the ANS consist of two sets of neurons arranged in series. **Preganglionic neurons** originate in the central nervous system and terminate in peripheral **ganglia**, where they synapse with **postganglionic neurons** innervating the target organs.

The sympathetic system

Sympathetic preganglionic neurons originate in the **intermedio-lateral** (IML) columns of the spinal cord. These neurons exit the spinal cord through ventral roots of segments T_1–L_2, and synapse with the postganglionic fibres in either *paravertebral* or *prevertebral* ganglia. The paravertebral ganglia are arranged in two sympathetic chains, one of which is shown in Fig. 27.1. These are located on either side of the spinal cord, and usually contain 22 or 23 ganglia. The prevertebral ganglia, shown to the left of the sympathetic chain, are diffuse structures which form part of the visceral autonomic plexuses of the abdomen and pelvis. The ganglionic neurotransmitter is **acetylcholine**, and it activates postganglionic **nicotinic cholinergic** receptors.

The postganglionic fibres terminate in the effector organs, where they release **norepinephrine**. Preganglionic sympathetic fibres also control the **adrenal medulla**, which releases **epinephrine** and norepinephrine into the blood. Under physiological conditions, the effect of neuronal norepinephrine release is more important than that of epinephrine and norepinephrine released by the adrenal medulla.

Epinephrine and norepinephrine are *catecholamines*, and activate **adrenergic** receptors in the effector organs. These receptors are *G-protein linked* and exist as three types:

1 α_1-**receptors** are linked to G_q and have subtypes α_{1A}, α_{1B} and α_{1D}. Epinephrine and norepinephrine activate α_1-receptors with similar potencies.

2 α_2-**receptors** are linked to $G_{i/o}$ and have subtypes α_{2A}, α_{2B} and α_{2C}. Epinephrine activates α_2-receptors more potently than does norepinephrine.

3 β-**receptors** are linked to G_s and have subtypes β_1, β_2 and β_3. Norepinephrine is more potent than epinephrine at β_1- and β_3-receptors, while epinephrine is more potent at β_2-receptors.

Effects on the heart

Catecholamines acting via cardiac β_1-**receptors** have positive inotropic and chronotropic effects via mechanisms described in Chapters 10 and 11. At rest, cardiac sympathetic nerves exert a tonic-accelerating influence on the sinoatrial node, which is, however, overshadowed in younger people by the opposite and dominant effect of parasympathetic vagal tone. Vagal tone decreases progressively with age, causing a rise in the resting heart rate as the sympathetic influence becomes more dominant.

Effects on the vasculature

At rest, vascular sympathetic nerves fire impulses at a rate of 1–2 impulses/s, thereby tonically vasoconstricting the arteries, arterioles and veins. Increasing activation of the sympathetic system causes further vasoconstriction. Vasoconstriction is mediated mainly by α_1-**receptors** on the vascular smooth muscle cells. The arterial system, particularly the arterioles, is more densely innervated by the sympathetic system than is the venous system. Sympathetic vasoconstriction is particularly marked in the splanchnic, renal, cutaneous and skeletal muscle vascular beds.

The vasculature also contains both β_1- and β_2-receptors, which when stimulated exert a *vasodilating* influence, especially in the *skeletal* and *coronary* circulations. These may play a limited role in dilating these vascular beds in response to epinephrine release, for example during mental stress. In some species, sympathetic *cholinergic* fibres innervate skeletal muscle blood vessels and cause vasodilatation during the defence reaction. A similar but minor role for such nerves in man has been proposed, but is unproven.

It is a common fallacy that the sympathetic nerves are always activated *en masse*. In reality, changes in sympathetic vasoconstrictor activity can be limited to certain regions (e.g. to the skin during thermoregulation). Similarly, a sympathetically mediated tachycardia occurs with no change in inotropy or vascular resistance during the Bainbridge reflex (see Chapter 26).

The parasympathetic system

The parasympathetic preganglionic neurons involved in regulating the heart have their cell bodies in the **nucleus ambiguus** and the **dorsal motor nucleus** of the medulla. Their axons run in the **vagus** nerve (cranial nerve X) and release acetylcholine onto nicotinic receptors on short postganglionic neurons originating in the cardiac plexus. These innervate the *sinoatrial (SAN)* and *atrioventricular nodes (AVN)* and the *atria*.

Effects on the heart

Basal acetylcholine release by vagal nerve terminals acts on muscarinic receptors to slow the discharge of the SAN. Increased vagal tone further decreases the heart rate and the speed of impulse conduction through the AVN and also decreases the force of atrial contraction when activated.

Effects on the vasculature

Although vagal slowing of the heart can decrease the blood pressure by lowering cardiac output, the parasympathetic system has no effect on total peripheral resistance, because it innervates only a limited number of vascular beds. In particular, activation of parasympathetic fibres in the pelvic nerve causes **erection** by vasodilating arterioles in the erectile tissue of the genitalia. Parasympathetic nerves also cause vasodilatation in the pancreas and salivary glands.

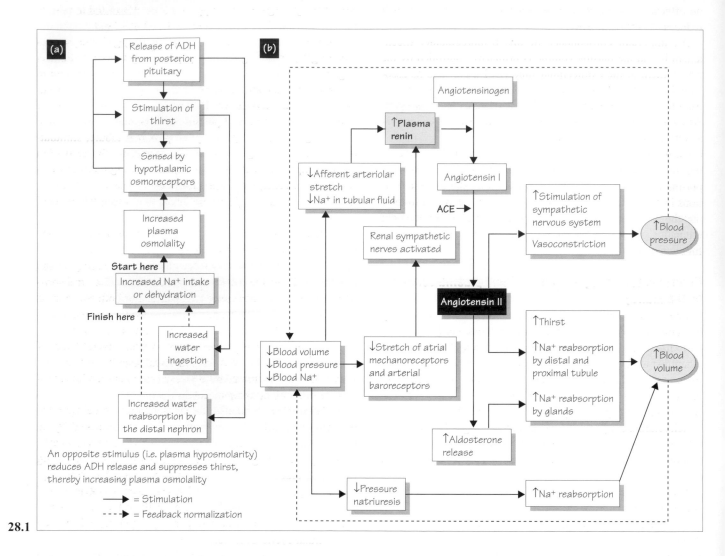

(a)

Release of ADH from posterior pituitary

Stimulation of thirst

Sensed by hypothalamic osmoreceptors

Increased plasma osmolality

Start here

Increased Na⁺ intake or dehydration

Finish here

Increased water ingestion

Increased water reabsorption by the distal nephron

An opposite stimulus (i.e. plasma hyposmolarity) reduces ADH release and suppresses thirst, thereby increasing plasma osmolality

⟶ = Stimulation

----▸ = Feedback normalization

(b)

Angiotensinogen

↑Plasma renin

↓Afferent arteriolar stretch
↓Na⁺ in tubular fluid

Angiotensin I

ACE →

Renal sympathetic nerves activated

↑Stimulation of sympathetic nervous system
Vasoconstriction

↑Blood pressure

Angiotensin II

↓Blood volume
↓Blood pressure
↓Blood Na⁺

↓Stretch of atrial mechanoreceptors and arterial baroreceptors

↑Thirst
↑Na⁺ reabsorption by distal and proximal tubule
↑Na⁺ reabsorption by glands

↑Blood volume

↑Aldosterone release

↓Pressure natriuresis

↑Na⁺ reabsorption

28.1

The baroreceptor system effectively minimizes short-term fluctuations in the arterial blood pressure. Over the longer term, however, the ability of the body to sustain a constant blood pressure depends on the maintenance of a *constant blood volume*. This dependency arises because alterations in the blood volume affect venous return and therefore cardiac output. Changes in cardiac output then ultimately lead to adaptive effects of the vasculature which increase peripheral resistance, and therefore blood pressure (see Chapter 36).

The volume of the blood is affected by changes in the total body contents of both Na⁺ and water. Both of these parameters are mainly controlled by the kidneys. The maintenance of a stable blood pressure therefore involves mechanisms that adjust renal excretion of sodium and water, so that the contents of both remain unchanged.

Plasma volume: the role of sodium and osmoregulation

Alterations in the water content of the body, caused for example by variations in fluid intake or perspiration, result in changes in the plasma **osmolality**. The osmolality of a solution is defined as the total concentration of osmotically active particles per kilogram of water.

Any deviation of plasma osmolality from its normal value of ~*300 mosmol/kg* is sensed by *hypothalamic osmoreceptors*, which activate the homeostatic feedback control system illustrated in Fig. 28.1(a). The osmoreceptors regulate both thirst and the release from the posterior pituitary gland of **antidiuretic hormone** (**ADH**, also **vasopressin**), a peptide which suppresses renal water excretion. For example, dehydration raises plasma osmolality. This results in an increased thirst, and also enhances the release of ADH. ADH acts on the distal nephron to increase its reabsorption of water, thereby reducing the loss of water in the urine. Both effects act to bring plasma osmolality back to its set point by restoring the water content of the body. The opposite effects are stimulated by an excess of body water, which reduces plasma osmolality.

An important consequence of this osmoregulatory mechanism is that the plasma volume is primarily controlled by the Na^+ content of the extracellular fluid (ECF). Na^+ and its associated anions Cl^- and HCO_3^- account for about 95% of the osmotic solute present in the ECF, of which the plasma is a part. Any change in the Na^+ content of the body (e.g. after eating a salty meal) will quickly affect plasma osmolality. This will cause the osmoregulatory system to readjust the body water content (and therefore the plasma volume) in order to restore the plasma osmolality. Under normal conditions, therefore, alterations in body Na^+ lead to changes in plasma volume. It follows that the maintenance of a stable plasma volume requires the tight regulation of the total body (and therefore ECF) Na^+ content, a function mainly carried out by the kidneys.

Control of total body Na^+ content and plasma volume by the kidneys

Studies in both animals and man have shown that the total body Na^+ content is maintained within narrow limits. The body apparently has a set point for total Na^+ content, and is able to sense when this deviations from this set point occur. This is referred to as 'sodium memory'. As shown in Fig. 28.1(b), changes in vascular volume, pressure and body Na^+ activate mechanisms which cause compensatory alterations in renal Na^+ excretion which return these parameters back to their original levels. Only effects of decreases in vascular volume and pressure are illustrated; however, increases in these parameters cause opposite compensatory responses.

Pressure natriuresis is an intrinsic renal homeostatic mechanism by which decreases in blood volume and pressure strongly inhibit diuresis and **natriuresis** (Na^+ excretion in the urine). Although the mechanisms of pressure natriuresis remain imperfectly understood, it is thought that decreases in renal perfusion pressure cause a fall in the hydrostatic pressure within the renal interstitium surrounding the proximal tubule. This promotes the reabsorption of fluid from the nephron, acting to restore the blood volume. Opposite effects occur during volume expansion.

The **renin–angiotensin–aldosterone system** responds to stimuli associated with reductions in vascular volume and pressure by inhibiting Na^+ excretion, increasing thirst, and causing vasoconstriction. **Renin** is a proteolytic enzyme stored in the *granular cells* of the renal juxtaglomerular apparatus. Renin release into the blood is increased by:

1 Activation of the baroreceptor reflex by a reduction of vascular pressure, which increases firing of sympathetic nerves innervating the granular cells.
2 Decreased atrial stretch/pressure, sensed by cardiac mechanoreceptors.
3 Decreased stretch of renal afferent arterioles caused by a fall in renal perfusion pressure.

4 The release of prostacyclin (PGI_2) by the *macula densa cells* of the early distal tubule. The macula densa cells, which form part of the juxtaglomerular apparatus, are stimulated to release PGI_2 by a fall in the NaCl content of the tubular fluid.

Once released, renin cleaves a plasma α_2-globulin, **angiotensinogen**, liberating the decapeptide **angiotensin I**. Plasma angiotensin I is then acted on by **angiotensin-converting enzyme** (ACE) on the surface of endothelial cells, giving rise to the octapeptide **angiotensin II**. Angiotensin II has a variety of effects, which raise blood pressure and volume. These include increasing Na^+ reabsorption by the proximal tubule, stimulating thirst, promoting ADH release, increasing the activation of the sympathetic nervous system, and causing a direct vasoconstriction. ACE, also called **kininase II**, has the additional function of breaking down bradykinin, a vasodilating local hormone.

Angiotensin II also promotes the release of the steroid hormone **aldosterone** from the zona glomerulosa cells of the adrenal cortex. Aldosterone increases Na^+ retention by acting on the principal cells of the distal nephron to enhance Na^+ reabsorption. It does so by increasing the synthesis of both Na^+ pumps in the basolateral membrane and Na^+ channels in the apical membrane of these cells. In addition, aldosterone conserves body Na^+ by enhancing its reabsorption from several types of glands, including the salivary and sweat glands. Aldosterone secretion is also increased by decreased stimulation of the atrial volume/pressure mechanoreceptors.

Atrial natriuretic peptide (ANP) is a 28-amino-acid peptide released from atrial myocytes when they are stretched by an increased atrial volume. ANP can cause both diuresis and natriuresis by increasing the glomerular filtration rate, decreasing renin and aldosterone secretion, and reducing Na^+ reabsorption throughout the nephron. ANP also dilates arterioles and increases capillary permeability. On a cellular level, ANP stimulates a membrane-associated guanylyl cyclase, raising the intracellular cyclic GMP concentration.

Recent studies in dogs suggest that pressure natriuresis and the renin–angiotensin–aldosterone system are of predominant and approximately equal importance in controlling total body Na^+, and therefore long-term blood pressure. ANP and other mechanisms such as changes in renal nitric oxide and prostaglandins seem to have a more limited role, and may be involved chiefly in the response to volume overload.

Antidiuretic hormone in volume regulation

Under emergency conditions, plasma volume is maintained at the expense of osmoregulation. For example, a fall in blood volume sensed by atrial pressure/stretch mechanoreceptors causes an increased ADH release, leading to water retention by the kidneys. In addition, the ADH system is rendered more sensitive to increases in plasma osmolality by a fall in vascular volume, so that ADH release is promoted even at normal plasma osmolality. Increases in plasma volume have the opposite effect on ADH release.

29 Cardiovascular effects of exercise

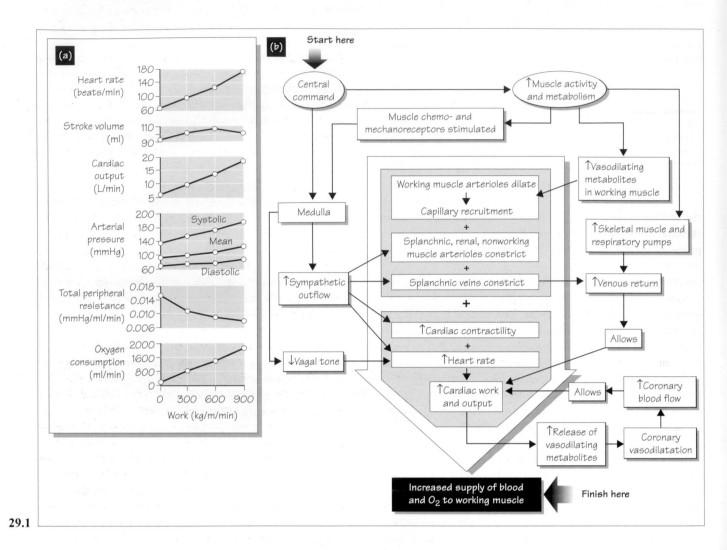

Figure 29.1(a) summarizes important cardiovascular adaptations which occur at increasing levels of dynamic (rhythmic) exercise, thereby allowing working muscles to be supplied with the increased amount of O_2 they require. By far the most important of these is an increase in cardiac output (CO), which rises almost linearly with the rate of muscle O_2 consumption (level of work) as a result of increases in both **heart rate** and to a lesser extent **stroke volume**. The heart rate is accelerated by a reduction in vagal tone, and by increases in sympathetic nerve firing and circulating catecholamines. The resulting stimulation of cardiac β-adrenoceptors increases stroke volume by *increasing myocardial contractility* and enabling more complete systolic emptying of the ventricles. CO is the limiting factor determining the maximum exercise capacity.

Table 29.1 shows that the increased CO is channelled mainly to the active muscles, which may receive 85% of CO, against about 15–20% at rest, and to the heart. This is caused by a profound arteriolar vasodilatation in these organs. Dilatation of terminal arterioles causes **capillary recruitment**, a large increase in the number of open capillaries, which shortens the diffusion distance between capillaries and muscle fibres. This, combined with increases in P_{CO_2}, temperature and acidity, promotes the release of O_2 from haemoglobin, allowing skeletal muscle to increase its O_2 extraction from the basal level of 25–30% to about 90% during maximal exercise.

Increased firing of sympathetic nerves and levels of circulating catecholamines constrict arterioles in the *splanchnic* and *renal* vascular beds, and in *nonexercising muscle*, reducing the bloodflow to these organs. Cutaneous bloodflow is also initially reduced. As core body temperature rises, however, cutaneous bloodflow increases as autonomically mediated vasodilatation occurs to promote cooling (see Chapter 24). With very strenuous exercise, cutaneous perfusion again falls as vasoconstriction diverts blood to the muscles. The increased CO necessitates a

Table 29.1 Cardiac output and regional blood flow in a sedentary man. Values are ml/min.

	Quiet standing	Exercise
Cardiac output	5900	24000
Blood flow to:		
Heart	250	1000
Brain	750	750
Active skeletal muscle	650	20850
Inactive skeletal muscle	650	300
Skin	500	500
Kidney, liver, gastrointestinal tract, etc.	3100	600

rise in venous return. This is enhanced by increased activity of skeletal muscle and respiratory pumps, and is also transiently promoted by splanchnic constriction, which reduces the capacitance of the venous system. Bloodflow to the crucial cerebral vasculature remains constant.

Vasodilatation of the skeletal and cutaneous vascular beds decreases total peripheral resistance. This is sufficient to balance the effect of the increased CO on diastolic blood pressure, which rises only slightly and may even fall, depending on the balance between skeletal muscle vasodilatation and splanchnic/renal vasoconstriction. Significant rises in the systolic and pulse pressures are, however, caused by the more rapid and forceful ejection of blood by the left ventricle, leading to some elevation of the mean arterial blood pressure.

Effects of exercise on plasma volume

Arteriolar dilatation in skeletal muscles increases capillary hydrostatic pressure, while capillary recruitment vastly increases the surface area of the microcirculation available to exchange fluid. These effects, coupled with a rise in interstitial osmolarity caused by an increased production of metabolites within the muscle fibres, lead via the Starling mechanism to *extravasation of fluid into muscles*. Taking into account also fluid losses caused by sweating, plasma volume may decrease by 15% during strenuous exercise. This fluid loss is partially compensated by enhanced fluid reabsorption in the vasoconstricted vascular beds, where capillary pressure decreases.

Regulation and coordination of the cardiovascular adaptation to exercise

In anticipation of exercise, and during its initial stages, a process termed **central command** (Fig. 29.1b, upper left) causes the cardiovascular adaptations necessary for increased effort. Impulses from the cerebral cortex act on the medulla to suppress vagal tone, thereby increasing the heart rate and CO. Central command is also thought to raise the set point of the baroreceptor reflex. This allows the blood pressure to be regulated around a higher set point, resulting in an increased sympathetic outflow which contributes to the rise in CO and causes

constriction of the splanchnic and renal circulations. An increase in circulating epinephrine also vasodilates skeletal muscle arterioles via β_2-receptors. The magnitude of these anticipatory effects increases in proportion to the degree of perceived effort.

As exercise continues, cardiovascular regulation by central command is supplemented by two further control systems which are activated and become crucial. These involve: (i) autonomic reflexes (Fig. 29.1b, left); and (ii) direct effects of metabolites generated locally in working skeletal and cardiac muscle (right).

Systemic effects mediated by autonomic reflexes

Nervous impulses originating mainly from receptors in working muscle which respond to contraction (mechanoreceptors) and locally generated metabolites and ischaemia (chemoreceptors) are carried to the CNS via afferent nerves. CNS autonomic control centres respond by suppressing vagal tone and causing graded increases in sympathetic outflow which are matched to the ongoing level of exercise. An increased release of epinephrine and norepinephrine from the adrenal glands causes plasma catecholamines to rise by as much as 10–20-fold.

Effects of local metabolites on muscle and heart

The autonomic reflexes described above are responsible for most of the cardiac and vasoconstricting adaptations to exercise. However, the marked vasodilatation of coronary and skeletal muscle arterioles is almost entirely caused by *local metabolites* generated in the heart and working skeletal muscle. This **metabolic hyperaemia** (Chapter 22) causes decreased vascular resistance and increased bloodflow. Capillary recruitment (see above) is an important consequence of metabolic hyperaemia.

Static exercises such as lifting and carrying involve maintained muscle contractions with no joint movement. This results in vascular compression and a decreased muscle bloodflow, leading to a build up of muscle metabolites. These activate muscle chemoreceptors, resulting in a **pressor reflex** involving *tachycardia*, and *increases* in *CO* and *TPR*. The resulting rise in blood pressure is much greater than in dynamic exercise causing the same rise in O_2 consumption.

Effects of training

Athletic training has effects on the cardiovascular system which improve delivery of O_2 to muscle cells, allowing them to work harder. The ventricular walls thicken and the cavities become larger, increasing the stroke volume from about 75 to 120 ml. The resting heart rate may fall as low as 45 beats/min, due to an increase in vagal tone, while the maximal rate remains near 180 beats/min. These changes allow CO, the crucial determinant of exercise capacity, to increase more during strenuous exercise, reaching levels of 35 L/min or more. TPR falls, in part due to a decreased sympathetic outflow. The capillary density of skeletal muscle increases, and the muscle fibres contain more mitochondria, promoting oxygen extraction and utilization.

30 Shock and haemorrhage

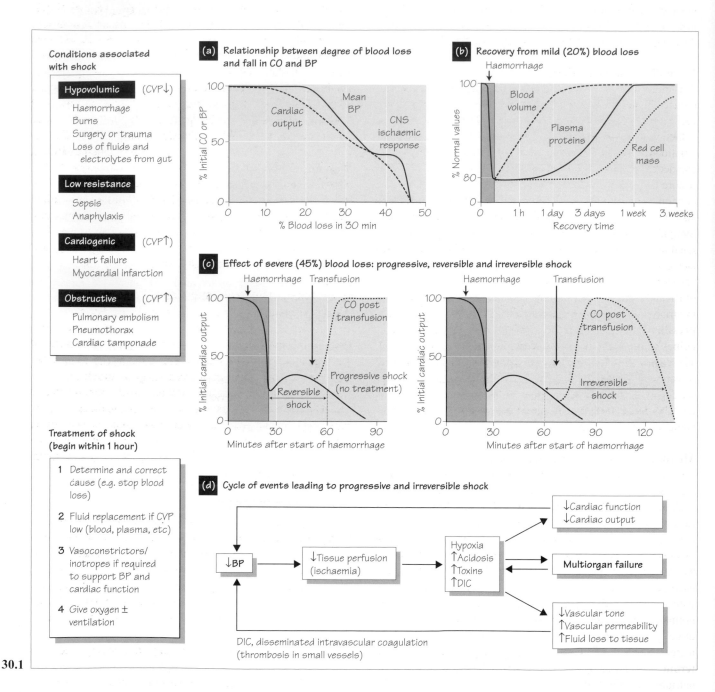

Conditions associated with shock

Hypovolumic (CVP↓)
- Haemorrhage
- Burns
- Surgery or trauma
- Loss of fluids and electrolytes from gut

Low resistance
- Sepsis
- Anaphylaxis

Cardiogenic (CVP↑)
- Heart failure
- Myocardial infarction

Obstructive (CVP↑)
- Pulmonary embolism
- Pneumothorax
- Cardiac tamponade

(a) Relationship between degree of blood loss and fall in CO and BP

(b) Recovery from mild (20%) blood loss

(c) Effect of severe (45%) blood loss: progressive, reversible and irreversible shock

(d) Cycle of events leading to progressive and irreversible shock

DIC, disseminated intravascular coagulation (thrombosis in small vessels)

Treatment of shock (begin within 1 hour)

1 Determine and correct cause (e.g. stop blood loss)

2 Fluid replacement if CVP low (blood, plasma, etc)

3 Vasoconstrictors/inotropes if required to support BP and cardiac function

4 Give oxygen ± ventilation

30.1

Cardiovascular or **circulatory shock** refers to an acute condition where there is a generalized inadequacy of bloodflow throughout the body. The patient appears pale, grey or cyanotic, with cold clammy skin, a weak, rapid pulse, and rapid shallow breathing. Urine output is reduced, and blood pressure (BP) is generally low. Conscious patients may suffer from intense thirst. Cardiovascular shock may be caused by a reduced blood volume (**hypovolumic shock**), profound vasodilatation (**low-resistance shock**), acute failure of the heart to maintain output (**cardiogenic shock**), or blockage of the cardiopulmonary circuit (e.g. pulmonary embolism).

Haemorrhagic shock

Blood loss (**haemorrhage**) is the commonest cause of shock. Loss of up to ~20% of total blood volume is unlikely to elicit shock in a fit person. If 20–30% of blood volume is lost, shock is normally induced and blood pressure may be depressed, although death is not common. Loss of 30–50% of volume, however, causes a profound reduction in BP and cardiac output (Fig. 30.1a), with severe shock which may become **irreversible** or **refractory** (see below). Severity is related to amount and rate of blood loss—a very rapid loss of 30% can be fatal, whereas 50% over 24 h may be survived. Above 50% death is generally inevitable.

Immediate compensation

The initial fall in BP is detected by the **baroreceptors**, and reduced bloodflow activates peripheral **chemoreceptors**. These cause a reflex increase in sympathetic and decrease in parasympathetic drive, with a subsequent increase in heart rate, venoconstriction (restores CVP) and vasoconstriction of the splanchnic, cutaneous, renal and skeletal muscle circulations which helps restore BP. Vasoconstriction leads to pallor, reduced urine production and lactic acidosis. Increased sympathetic discharge also results in sweating, and characteristic clammy skin. Sympathetic vasoconstriction of the renal artery plus reduced renal artery pressure stimulates the **renin–angiotensin system** (see Chapter 28), and production of **angiotensin II**, a powerful vasoconstrictor. This plays an important role in the recovery of BP and stimulates thirst. In more severe blood loss, reduction in atrial stretch receptor output stimulates production of **vasopressin** (antidiuretic hormone, **ADH**) and adrenal production of **epinephrine**, both of which contribute to vasoconstriction. These initial mechanisms may prevent any significant fall in BP or cardiac output following moderate blood loss, even though the degree of shock may be serious. If BP falls below 50 mmHg the **CNS ischaemic response** is activated, with powerful sympathetic activation (Fig. 30.1a).

Medium- and long-term mechanisms

The vasoconstriction and/or fall in BP decreases capillary hydrostatic pressure, resulting in fluid movement from the interstitium back into the vasculature (see Chapter 20). This 'internal transfusion' may increase blood volume by ~0.5 L and takes hours to develop. Increased glucose production by the liver may contribute by raising plasma and interstitial fluid osmolarity, thus drawing water from intracellular compartments. This process results in haemodilution, and patients with severe shock often present with a reduced haematocrit. Fluid volume is brought back to normal over days by increased fluid intake (thirst), decreased urine production (**oliguria**) due to renal vasoconstriction, increased Na^+ reabsorption caused by the production of **aldosterone** (stimulated by angiotensin II) and a fall in **ANP** (atrial natriuretic peptide), and increased water reabsorption caused by vasopressin (Fig. 30.1b). The liver replaces plasma proteins within a week, and haematocrit returns to normal within 6 weeks due to stimulation of **erythropoiesis** (Fig. 30.1b; see Chapter 6).

Other responses to haemorrhage: *Increased ventilation* due to reduced flow through **chemoreceptors** (carotid body) and/or acidosis; *decreased blood coagulation time* due an increase in platelets and fibrinogen that occurs in minutes (see Chapter 7); and *increased white cell (neutrophil) count* after 2–5 h.

Complications and irreversible (refractory) shock

When blood loss exceeds 30%, cardiac output may temporarily improve before continuing to decline (**progressive shock**; Fig. 30.1c). This is due to a vicious circle initiated by circulatory failure and tissue hypoxia/ischaemia, leading to acidosis, toxin release and eventually **multiorgan failure**, including **depression of cardiac muscle function**, acute respiratory distress syndrome (**ARDS**), **renal failure**, disseminated intravascular coagulation (**DIC**), **hepatic failure** and damage to **intestinal mucosa**. Increased vascular permeability further decreases blood volume due to fluid loss into the tissues, and vascular tone is depressed. These complications lead to further tissue damage, impairment of tissue perfusion and gas exchange (Fig. 30.1d). Rapid treatment (e.g. transfusion) is essential; after 1 h ('*the golden hour*') mortality increases sharply if the patient is still in shock, as transfusion and vasoconstrictor drugs may then cause only a temporary respite before cardiac output falls irrevocably. This is called **irreversible** or **refractory** shock (Fig. 30.1c), and is primarily related to irretrievable damage to the heart.

Other types of hypovolumic shock

Severe burns result in a loss of plasma in exudate from damaged tissue. As red cells are not lost, there is **haemoconcentration**, which will increase blood viscosity. Treatment of burns-related shock therefore involves infusion of plasma rather than whole blood. **Traumatic and surgical shock** can occur after major injury or surgery. Although partly due to external blood loss, blood and plasma can also be lost into the tissues, and there may be dehydration. **Other conditions** include severe diarrhoea or vomiting and loss of Na^+ (e.g. **cholera**) with a consequent reduction in blood volume even if water is given, unless electrolytes are replenished.

Low-resistance shock

Unlike hypovolumic shock, low-resistance shock may present with warm skin due to profound peripheral vasodilatation.

Septic shock is caused by a profound vasodilatation due to endotoxins released by infecting bacteria, partly via induction of inducible nitric oxide synthase (see Chapter 23). Capillary permeability and cardiac function may be impaired, with consequent loss of fluid to the tissues and depressed cardiac output.

Anaphylactic shock is a rapidly developing and life-threatening condition resulting from presentation of antigen to a sensitized individual, e.g. bee stings or peanut allergy. A severe **allergic reaction** may result, with release of large amounts of histamine. This causes profound vasodilatation, and increased microvasculature permeability, leading to protein and fluid loss to tissues (oedema). Rapid treatment with antihistamines and glucocorticoids is necessary, but immediate application of a vasoconstrictor (epinephrine) may be required to save the patient's life.

31 Risk factors for cardiovascular disease

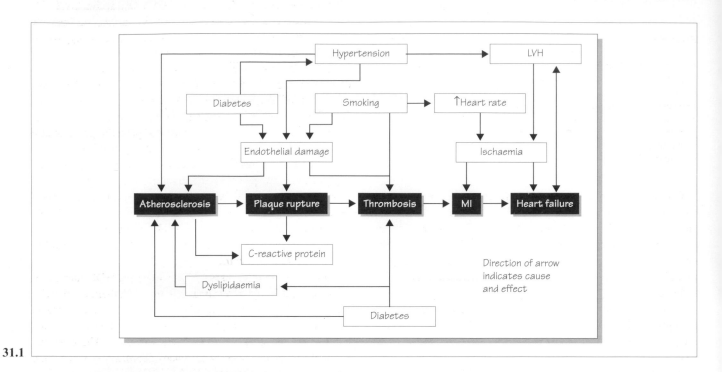

31.1

Cardiovascular risk factors are markers, the presence or levels of which correlate with the future probability of cardiovascular disease (CVD) and/or death. Risk factors are usually causes or promotors of CVD, but in other cases simply indicate that subclinical (i.e. as yet symptomless) CVD is already likely to be present. Table 31.1 presents an abbreviated summary of the impact of major risk factors on coronary heart disease as determined by the Framingham Heart Study.

Risk factors can be **fixed** or **modifiable**. Fixed risk factors include *age*, *male sex* and *family history of CVD*. Modifiable risk factors, including *smoking*, *dyslipidaemias*, *hypertension*, *diabetes mellitus*, *obesity* and *physical inactivity*, can be eliminated or ameliorated by lifestyle alteration and/or pharmacological therapy. This approach has been shown to reduce the occurrence and severity of CVD, and is particularly justified because overt CVD is typically both irreversible and ultimately lethal. Patients often have multiple modifiable risk factors, in which case all of these should be simultaneously targeted.

Figure 31.1 illustrates the main mechanisms by which major risk factors are thought to promote the development of atherosclerosis and its most important consequence, **coronary heart disease**. Specific aspects of these processes are described in greater detail in Chapters 33, 34, 37, 38, 41 and 44.

Modifiable risk factors

Dyslipidaemias are a heterogeneous group of conditions characterized by abnormal levels of one or more **lipoproteins**. Lipoproteins are blood-borne particles that contain cholesterol

and other lipids. They function to transfer lipids between the intestines, liver and other organs (see Chapter 33).

Dyslipidaemias involving excessive plasma concentrations of **low density lipoprotein**, or **LDL**, are associated with rises in plasma cholesterol levels, because LDL contains 70% of total plasma cholesterol. As the level of plasma cholesterol rises, particularly above 240 mg/dl (6.2 mmol/L), there is a progressive increase in the risk of CVD due to the attendant rise in LDL levels. LDL plays a pivotal role in causing atherosclerosis because it can be converted to an oxidized form, which damages the vascular wall (see Chapter 34). Drugs that lower plasma LDL (and therefore oxidized LDL) slow the progression of atherosclerosis and reduce the occurrence of CVD. Elevated levels of **lipoprotein (a)**, a form of LDL containing the unique protein *apo(a)*, have been reported to confer additional cardiovascular risk. Apo(a) contains a structural component closely resembling plasminogen, and it may inhibit fibrinolysis (see Chapter 7) by competing with plasminogen for endogenous activators.

Conversely, the risk of CVD is *inversely* related to the plasma concentration of **high density lipoprotein (HDL)**, possibly because HDL functions to remove cholesterol from body tissues, and may act to inhibit lipoprotein oxidation. The ratio of total : HDL cholesterol is therefore a better predictor of risk than cholesterol levels *per se*. Low HDL levels often coexist with high levels of plasma *triglycerides*, which are also correlated with CVD. This is probably due to the atherogenicity of the triglyceride-rich **very low density lipoprotein (VLDL)** and **intermediate density lipoprotein (IDL)**.

Table 31.1 Major modifiable risk factors: effects on the risk of coronary heart disease in men and women aged 35–64 years.

Risk factors	Age-adjusted relative risk*	
	Men	Women
Cholesterol > 240 mg/dl	1.9	1.8
Hypertension > 140/90 mmHg	2.0	2.2
Diabetes	1.5	3.7
Left ventricular hypertrophy	3.0	4.6
Smoking	1.5	1.1

* Indicates relative risk for individuals with a given factor vs those without it.

C-reactive protein (CRP): Atherosclerosis can be viewed as a chronic low-grade inflammation which is localized to certain sites of the vascular wall. This causes the release into the plasma of numerous inflammatory mediators and related substances. One of these, the acute phase reactant C-reactive protein, is particularly well suited for use as a marker of atherosclerosis, as it is stable and can be quickly and easily measured. Many epidemiological studies have shown that high basal levels of CRP are strongly predictive of future CVD. Importantly, high CRP levels are predictive of cardiovascular disease even in those with low LDL.

In addition to being predictive of future CVD in those who are as yet symptomless, CRP levels are often highly elevated following a heart attack or other acute coronary syndrome (see Chapter 38). In this situation, the extent of CRP elevation is correlated with an adverse short-term prognosis. This is likely to occur because atherosclerotic lesions in which an intense inflammatory reaction is occurring are probably more prone to rupture and cause coronary artery occlusion (see Chapter 38).

Hypertension, defined as a blood pressure above 140/90 mmHg, occurs in ~25% of the population. Hypertension promotes atherogenesis, probably by damaging the endothelium and causing other deleterious effects on the walls of large arteries. Hypertension damages blood vessels of the brain and kidneys, increasing the risk of stroke and renal failure. The higher cardiac workload imposed by the increased arterial pressure also causes a thickening of the left ventricular wall. This process, termed **left ventricular hypertrophy (LVH)** is both a cause and harbinger of more serious cardiovascular damage. LVH predisposes the myocardium to arrhythmias and ischaemia, and is a major contributor to heart failure, myocardial infarction and sudden death.

Physical inactivity promotes CVD via multiple mechanisms. Low fitness is associated with reduced plasma HDL, higher levels of blood pressure and insulin resistance, and **obesity**, itself a CVD risk factor. Studies show that a moderate to high level of fitness is associated with a halving of CVD mortality.

Diabetes mellitus is a metabolic disease present in approximately 5% of the population. Diabetics either lack the hormone *insulin* entirely, or become resistant to its actions. The latter condition, which usually develops in adulthood, is termed noninsulin-dependent diabetes (NIDDM), and accounts for 95% of diabetics. Diabetes causes progressive damage to both the microvasculature and larger arteries over many years. Approximately 75% of diabetics eventually die from CVD.

There is evidence that NIDDM patients have both endothelial damage and increased levels of oxidized LDL. Both effects may be a result of mechanisms associated with the hyperglycaemia characteristic of this condition. Also, blood coagulability is increased in NIDDM because of elevated plasminogen activator inhibitor 1 (PAI-1) and increased platelet aggregability.

A set of cardiovascular risk factors including high plasma triglycerides, low plasma HDL, hypertension, elevated plasma glucose and obesity (particularly abdominal) are often associated with each other. This combination of risk factors is closely linked to, and could arise as a result of, **insulin resistance**. Individuals with three or more of these risk factors are said to have **metabolic syndrome**.

Tobacco smoking causes CVD by lowering HDL, increasing blood coagulability and damaging the endothelium, thereby promoting atherosclerosis. In addition, nicotine-induced cardiac stimulation and a carbon monoxide-mediated reduction of the oxygen-carrying capacity of the blood also occur. These effects, coupled with an increased occurrence of coronary spasm, set the stage for cardiac ischaemia and myocardial infarction. Epidemiological evidence suggests that CVD risk is not reduced with low tar cigarettes.

Fixed risk factors
Family history of CVD
Numerous epidemiological surveys have shown the existence of a familial predisposition to CVD. This arises in part because many CVD risk factors (e.g. hypertension) have a *multifactorial genetic basis* (are due to multiple abnormal genes interacting with environmental influences). Additional deleterious genetic influences are also probably involved, because the familial predisposition remains if epidemiological data are corrected for known risk factors. For example, the angiotensin-converting enzyme (ACE) gene can exist in two forms, characterized by the insertion/deletion of a 287-base pair DNA segment within intron 16. Those homozygous for the deletion polymorphism have higher plasma ACE concentrations, which may modestly increase the risk of suffering myocardial infarction.

Male sex
Middle-aged women are much less likely than men to develop CVD. This difference progressively narrows after the menopause, and is mainly oestrogen mediated. Oestrogen's potentially beneficial actions include acting as an antioxidant, lowering LDL and raising HDL, stimulating the expression and activity of nitric oxide synthase, causing vasodilatation and increasing the production of plasminogen.

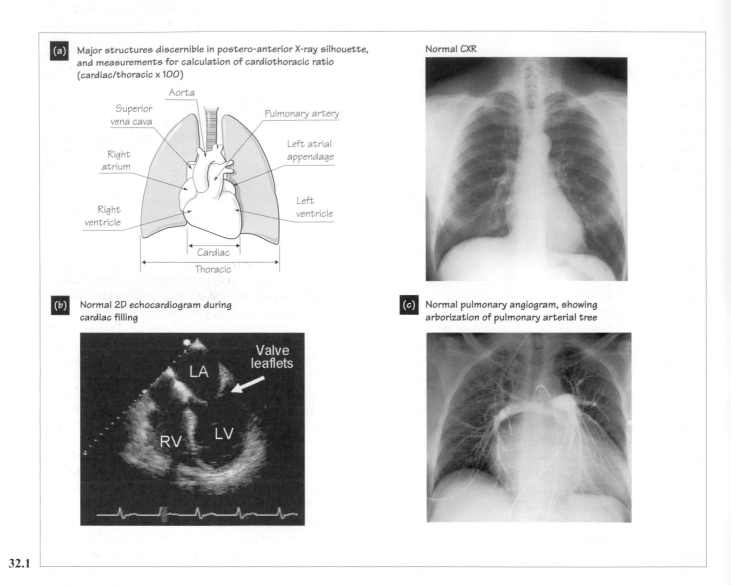

(a) Major structures discernible in postero-anterior X-ray silhouette, and measurements for calculation of cardiothoracic ratio (cardiac/thoracic x 100)

Aorta
Superior vena cava
Pulmonary artery
Left atrial appendage
Right atrium
Right ventricle
Left ventricle
Cardiac
Thoracic

Normal CXR

(b) Normal 2D echocardiogram during cardiac filling

Valve leaflets
LA
RV
LV

(c) Normal pulmonary angiogram, showing arborization of pulmonary arterial tree

32.1

General investigations

The arterial pulse, electrocardiogram (ECG) and heart sounds are dealt with in Chapters 13 and 16.

Blood pressure

Measurements are made using a **sphygmomanometer**. This consists of an inflatable cuff around the upper arm over the brachial artery, connected to a pressure gauge. The cuff is inflated until its pressure is greater than systolic pressure, at which point the arteries are compressed and the radial pulse disappears. A stethoscope is placed over the artery just below the cuff, and the cuff pressure is slowly reduced. When the pressure falls to the level of the systolic blood pressure, clear sounds are heard (**Korotkoff sounds**). These are due to turbulence as blood is forced through the partially occluded artery. As the cuff

pressure declines, the Korotkoff sounds become suddenly muffled, and then disappear completely. This cuff pressure is generally taken as diastolic pressure, as it is easiest to recognize. Sometimes the sounds disappear then reappear between the systolic and diastolic pressures, and care should be taken not to confuse these changes with their final disappearance.

Jugular venous pressure

Pressure in the internal jugular vein provides an estimate of right atrial pressure (see Chapter 13). Jugular venous pressure (JVP) is measured in patients positioned at an angle of 30–60°, and is taken as the vertical height between the manubriosternal angle and the point at which the vein collapses, i.e. the height of the venous column at end-expiration. JVP is normally less than 3 cm, but is increased when central venous pressure (CVP) is raised, e.g. **right heart failure**. *Tricuspid regurgitation* (back-flow during systole) causes a very large pulse.

X-rays (chest radiography)

The chest X-ray (CXR) is an essential diagnostic tool. The initial CXR is taken in the postero-anterior (PA) direction. Figure 32.1(a) shows diagrammatically the major structures in which gross abnormalities can be detected, such as enlargement of the heart chambers and major vessels, and a normal PA CXR. Heart size and **cardiothoracic ratio** (size of heart relative to thoracic cavity) can also be estimated. This ratio is normally < 50%, except in neonates, infants and athletes, but may be greatly increased in heart failure (see Chapter 44). Calcification due to tissue damage and necrosis may be detected by CXR if significant. Enlargement of the main pulmonary arteries coupled with pruning of the peripheral arteries suggests pulmonary hypertension, whereas haziness of the lung fields is indicative of pulmonary venous hypertension and fluid accumulation in the tissues.

Echocardiography and Doppler ultrasound

Echocardiography can be used to detect enlarged hearts and abnormal cardiac movement, and to estimate the ejection fraction. An ultrasound pulse of ~2.5 MHz is generated by a piezo-electric transmitter–receiver on the chest wall, and is reflected back by internal structures. As sound travels through fluid at a known velocity, the time taken between transmission and reception is a measure of distance. This allows a picture of internal structure to be built up. In an M-mode echocardiogram the transmitter remains static, and the trace shows changes in reflections with time. In 2D echocardiograms the transmitter scans backwards and forwards, so that a two-dimensional picture is built up (Fig. 32.1b).

Sound reflected back from a moving target shows a shift in frequency, e.g. if the target is moving towards the source, the frequency is increased. This **Doppler** effect can be used to calculate the *velocity* of blood movement from the frequency shift in the ultrasound pulse caused by reflection from red cells, and the *pressure gradient* across obstructions from the Bernoulli equation: $P = 4 \times (velocity)^2$. Bloodflow can be calculated if the cross-sectional area of the vessel is estimated using echocardiography.

Cardiac catheterization and angiography

Radiopaque catheters (opaque to X-rays) are introduced into the heart or blood vessels via peripheral veins or arteries. Catheters with small balloons at the tip (**Swan–Ganz** catheters) assist placement from the venous side as the tip moves with the flow. Placement can be ascertained from the pressure wave-form and X-rays. Catheters are used for measurement of pressures or cardiac output, **angiography**, or to take samples for estimating metabolites and Po_2. Left atrial pressure cannot be measured directly as it requires access via the mitral valve. Instead, a Swan–Ganz catheter is passed through the right heart, and is wedged in a distal pulmonary artery. As there is thus no flow through that artery, the pressure is the same throughout the capillaries to the pulmonary vein. This **pulmonary wedge pressure** is an estimate of left atrial pressure.

Angiography: A catheter is used to introduce a radiopaque **contrast medium** into the cardiac chambers, coronary or pulmonary arteries (Fig. 32.1c). This allows direct visualization of the blood and vessels with X-rays, and can be used to examine cardiac pumping function and to locate blockages (e.g. emboli) in the coronary and pulmonary circulations, amongst others.

Imaging

Advances in medical imaging techniques have provided several powerful diagnostic aids, of particular use in cardiac disease.

Nuclear imaging: Radiopharmaceuticals introduced into the heart or circulation are detected by a gamma camera, and their distribution (depending on type) can be used to measure or detect cardiac muscle perfusion, damage and function. 3D information can be obtained in a similar fashion using single photon computed tomography (**SPECT**). The most common tracers used are thallium-201 (^{201}Tl), and technetium-99 (^{99m}Tc)-labelled sestamibi (a large synthetic molecule of the isonitrile family), which are distributed according to bloodflow and taken up by living cardiac muscle cells. These therefore show up brightly immediately after infusion; ischaemic and infarcted areas remain dark because of poor perfusion. Whereas over time ^{201}Tl will redistribute into ischaemic areas as well, ^{99m}Tc-sestamibi will not, so a delayed ^{201}Tl image will show infarcted areas only. This is useful for determining savable areas of the heart prior to angioplasty or coronary bypass. ^{99m}Tc, however, has a higher photon energy and shorter half-life, allowing lower radio-nucleotide doses with better images. It is therefore better for SPECT, and the higher energy allows **gated acquisition** (sequential images taken during a cardiac cycle), and evaluation of resting left and right ventricular function in combination with either resting or exercise myocardial perfusion.

Magnetic resonance imaging (MRI): Radiofrequency stimulation of hydrogen atoms held in a high magnetic field emits energy, which can be used to generate a high fidelity image that reflects tissue density. MRI is useful for the location of masses and malformations, including aneurysms. It is entirely non-invasive and uses no damaging radiations.

33 Hyperlipidaemias

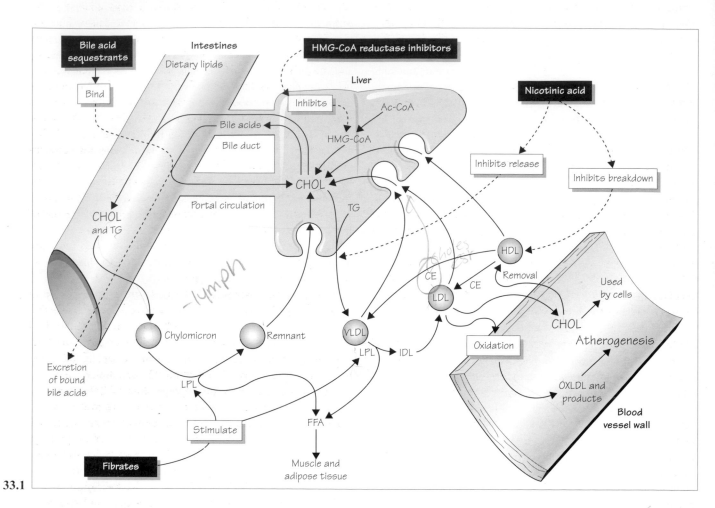

33.1

All cells require **lipids** (fats) to synthesize membranes and provide energy. Lipids are transported in the blood as **lipoproteins**. These small particles consist of a core of **triglycerides** and **cholesteryl esters**, surrounded by a coat of **phospholipids**, **cholesterol** and proteins, termed **apolipoproteins** or **apoproteins**. Apoproteins stabilize the lipoprotein particles and help target specific types of lipoproteins to various tissues. **Hyperlipidaemias** are abnormalities of lipoprotein levels, which promote the development of *atherosclerosis* (see Chapter 34) and *coronary heart disease* (CHD) (see Chapters 37–39).

Lipoproteins and lipid transport

Figure 33.1 illustrates pathways of lipid transport in the body. The **exogenous** pathway (left side of the figure) delivers ingested lipids to the body tissues and liver. Ingested triglycerides and cholesterol are combined with apoproteins in the intestinal mucosa to form **chylomicrons**. Passing into the bloodstream via the lymphatic system, chylomicrons bind to the capillary endothelium in muscle and adipose tissue. Here, their triglycerides are hydrolysed by the enzyme **lipoprotein lipase**

(LPL), yielding fatty acids which enter the tissues. The liver takes up the residual **chylomicron remnants**. These are broken down to yield cholesterol, which the liver also synthesizes. The rate-limiting enzyme in cholesterol synthesis is **hydroxymethylglutaryl coenzyme A reductase** (HMG-CoA reductase). The liver uses cholesterol to make bile acids and membrane components.

The **endogenous** pathway cycles lipids between the liver and peripheral tissues. The liver forms **very low density lipoproteins** (VLDLs), consisting mainly of triglycerides, with some cholesterol. VLDL triglycerides are hydrolysed by LPL, providing fatty acids to body tissues. As it is progressively drained of triglycerides, VLDL becomes **intermediate density lipoprotein** (IDL) and then **low density lipoprotein** (LDL), losing all of its apoproteins except for **apo B100** in the process. Most of the LDL, which contains mainly cholesteryl esters, is taken up by the liver. The remaining LDL serves to distribute cholesterol to the peripheral tissues. Cells regulate their cholesterol uptake by expressing more *LDL receptors* (which bind LDL via its apo B100) when their cholesterol requirement increases.

Cholesterol is removed from tissues by **high density lipoprotein** (HDL), which is initially assembled in the plasma from lipids and apoproteins (particularly **apo A1**) lost by other lipoproteins. It accumulates cholesterol from cell membranes and transfers it (as cholesterol esters) to VLDL, IDL and LDL, which return it to the liver.

Hyperlipidaemias: types and treatments

Primary hyperlipidaemias are caused by genetic abnormalities affecting apoproteins, apoprotein receptors or enzymes involved in lipoprotein metabolism. *Secondary* hyperlipidaemias are caused by conditions or drugs (e.g. diabetes, renal disease, alcohol abuse, thiazide diuretics) affecting lipoprotein metabolism. Diets high in saturated fats also cause hypercholesterolaemia, probably by decreasing hepatic lipoprotein clearance. The **Frederickson/WHO classification** identifies six hyperlipidaemic phenotypes. Type IIa involves **hypercholesterolaemia** with elevated LDL-cholesterol but normal triglycerides. Types I, IV and V involve mainly **hypertriglyceridaemia**, in which VLDL and/or chylomicron levels are raised. In **hypercholesterolaemia with hypertriglyceridaemia** (types IIb and III) both cholesterol and triglycerides are elevated.

The treatment of hyperlipidaemias aims to lower LDL-cholesterol and/or triglycerides, and to raise HDL-cholesterol. Patients with CHD or multiple cardiovascular risk factors require an especially aggressive normalization of lipid levels. Therapy reduces the risk of CHD, and can cause the *regression* of existing atherosclerotic lesions. Desirable total and LDL serum cholesterol levels are less than 200 mg/dl (5.2 mmol/L) and 130 mg/dl (3.4 mmol/L), respectively. The National Cholesterol Education Program in the United States suggests that lipid-lowering therapy is appropriate for anyone whose LDL-cholesterol is above 160 mg/dl (4.1 mmol/L), and for those with two or more risk factors if their serum LDL-cholesterol is above 130 mg/dl (3.4 mmol/L). For patients with CHD, diabetes or a 10-year risk of developing CHD of 20%, therapy is recommended if LDL-cholesterol is more than 100 mg/dl (2.6 mmol/L).

Treatment often begins with a low fat, high carbohydrate diet. If this fails to normalize hyperlipidaemia adequately after 3 months, therapy with a lipid-lowering drug is considered. Most of those with high cholesterol are treated with 'statins', since these have been repeatedly shown to reduce CHD and the mortality it causes. It is increasingly appreciated, however, that in addition to elevated LDL, high levels of triglycerides (reflected by high VLDL) and low levels of HDL promote the development of atherosclerosis. This combination of factors is common in those with *metabolic syndrome*, and the use with statins of 'fibrates' and nicotinic acid, which cause large increases in HDL levels, will probably increase in these individuals.

HMG-CoA reductase inhibitors or 'statins' include **simvastatin**, **lovastatin**, **pravastatin**, **fluvastatin**, **mevastatin** and **atorvastatin**. The West of Scotland Coronary Prevention Study (WOSCOPS) reported in 1995 that treatment of middle-aged men with high cholesterol but no history of myocardial infarction (MI) using pravastatin reduced the incidence of MI or death from cardiovascular disease by 31% over a 5-year period. Remarkably, the AFCAPS/TexCAPS trial reported in 1998 that over a similar period lovastatin reduced the incidence of first MI by 40% in individuals with low HDL but *average* cholesterol levels. Statins reduce hepatic synthesis of cholesterol, causing an upregulation of hepatic receptors for B and E apoproteins. This increases the clearance of LDL, IDL and VLDL from the plasma. Statins also increase plasma HDL levels by an unknown mechanism. There is increasing evidence that the statins also enhance nitric oxide release, possibly by activating the PI3K/Akt pathway (see Chapter 23), thereby reducing the coronary artery vasoconstriction that often contributes to acute coronary syndromes (see Chapter 38). Serious adverse effects associated with the use of statins are very rare. They include *hepatotoxicity* and *rhabdomyolysis* (destruction of skeletal muscle), the risk of which is increased with concomitant use of nicotinic acid or a fibric acid derivative. **Rosuvastatin** is a new drug, currently awaiting regulatory approval, which causes a greater reduction in LDL levels than do other statins.

Bile acid sequestrants: Bile acids are synthesized from cholesterol in the liver, and cycle between the liver and intestine (enterohepatic recirculation). **Cholestyramine** and **cholestipol** are exchange resins that bind and trap bile acids in the intestine, increasing their excretion. This enhances hepatic bile acid synthesis and cholesterol utilization. The resulting depletion of hepatic cholesterol causes an upregulation of LDL receptors, increasing the clearance of LDL-cholesterol from the plasma. The bile acid sequestrants cause little systemic toxicity because they are not absorbed. They are, however, taken in large amounts (e.g. up to 30 g/day), and cause gastrointestinal side effects such as nausea, diarrhoea and reflux oesophagitis.

Nicotinic acid (niacin) is a B vitamin that has lipid-lowering effects at high doses. It inhibits the synthesis and release of VLDL by the liver. Because VLDL gives rise to IDL and LDL, plasma levels of these lipoproteins also fall. Conversely, HDL levels rise as a result of decreased breakdown. Nicotinic acid can cause a number of adverse effects, including hepatotoxicity, palpitations, impairment of glucose tolerance, hyperuricaemia, hypotension and amblyopia. Most patients experience flushing when starting nicotinic acid therapy. This is caused by vasodilatation, which is secondary to prostaglandin release from the endothelium. This can be prevented by nonsteroidal antiinflammatory drugs.

Fibric acid derivatives ('fibrates') include **gemfibrazole**, **clofibrate**, **bezafibrate**, **ciprofibrate** and **fenofibrate**. These stimulate the activity of lipoprotein lipase, thereby reducing VLDL triglycerides by increasing their hydrolysis. They also promote changes in LDL composition, which render it less atherogenic, and enhance fibrolysis. Fibrates are mainly used with types IIb and III hyperlipidaemias. They cause mild gastrointestinal disorders in 5–10% of patients, and can potentially cause muscle toxicity and renal failure if combined with HMG-CoA reductase inhibitors or excessive alcohol use.

34 Atherosclerosis

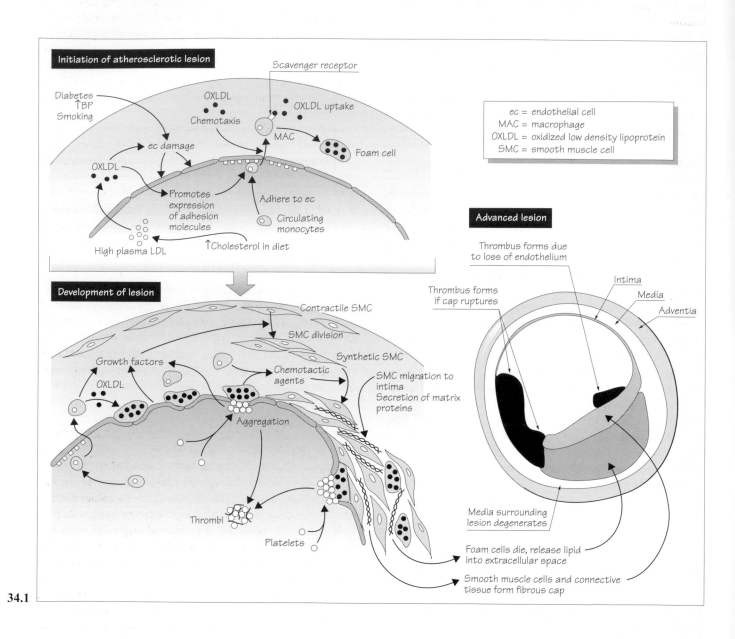

Initiation of atherosclerotic lesion

Scavenger receptor

Diabetes
↑BP
Smoking

OXLDL

OXLDL uptake

Chemotaxis

MAC

Foam cell

ec damage

OXLDL

Promotes expression of adhesion molecules

Adhere to ec

Circulating monocytes

High plasma LDL

↑Cholesterol in diet

ec = endothelial cell
MAC = macrophage
OXLDL = oxidized low density lipoprotein
SMC = smooth muscle cell

Advanced lesion

Thrombus forms due to loss of endothelium

Intima
Media
Adventia

Thrombus forms if cap ruptures

Development of lesion

Contractile SMC

SMC division

Growth factors

Synthetic SMC

OXLDL

Chemotactic agents

SMC migration to intima
Secretion of matrix proteins

Aggregation

Thrombi

Platelets

Media surrounding lesion degenerates

Foam cells die, release lipid into extracellular space

Smooth muscle cells and connective tissue form fibrous cap

34.1

Atherosclerosis is a disease of the larger arteries. It begins in childhood with localized accumulations of lipid within the arterial intima, termed **fatty streaks**. By middle age some of these develop into **atherosclerotic plaques**, focal lesions where the arterial wall is grossly abnormal. Plaques may be several centimetres across, and are most common in the *aorta*, the *coronary* and *internal carotid arteries*, and the *circle of Willis*. An advanced atherosclerotic plaque, illustrated on the right of the diagram, demonstrates several features.

1 The arterial wall is focally thickened by intimal smooth muscle cell proliferation and the deposition of fibrous connective tissue, forming a hard **fibrous cap**. This projects into the vascular lumen, restricting the flow of blood, and often causes ischaemia in the tissue region served by the artery.

2 A soft pool of extracellular lipid and cell debris accumulates beneath the fibrous cap (*athera* is Greek for gruel or porridge). This weakens the arterial wall, so that the fibrous cap may fissure or tear away. As a result, blood enters the lesions and **thrombi** (blood clots) are formed. These thrombi, or the material leaking from the ruptured lesion, may be carried to the upstream vascular bed to *embolize* (plug) smaller vessels. A larger thrombus may totally occlude (block) the artery at the site of the lesion. This causes myocardial infarction or stroke if it occurs in a coronary or cerebral artery, respectively.

3 The endothelium over the lesion is partially or completely lost. This can lead to ongoing formation of thrombi, causing intermittent flow occlusion as in unstable angina.

4 The medial smooth muscle layer under the lesion degenerates. This weakens the vascular wall, which may distend and eventually rupture (an **aneurysm**). Aneurysms are especially common in the abdominal aorta.

Atherosclerotic arteries may also demonstrate spasms or reduced vasodilatation. This worsens the restriction of the bloodflow and promotes thrombus formation (Chapters 38, 41).

Pathogenesis of atherosclerosis

The risk of developing atherosclerosis is in part genetically determined. The incidence of clinical consequences of atherosclerosis such as ischaemic heart disease rises with age, especially after age 40. Atherosclerosis is much more common in men than in women. This difference is probably due to a protective effect of oestrogen, and progressively disappears after menopause. Important risk factors that predispose towards atherosclerosis include smoking, hypertension, diabetes and high serum cholesterol.

The most widely accepted hypothesis for the pathogenesis of atherosclerosis proposes that it is initiated by *endothelial injury or dysfunction*. Plaques tend to develop in areas of variable haemodynamic sheer stress (e.g. where arteries branch or bifurcate). The endothelium is especially vulnerable to damage at such sites, as evidenced by increased endothelial cell turnover and permeability. Endothelial dysfunction promotes the adhesion of **monocytes**, white blood cells which burrow beneath the endothelial monolayer and become **macrophages**. Macrophages normally play an important role during inflammation, the body's response to injury and infection. They do so by acting as scavenger cells to remove dead cells and foreign material, and also by subsequently releasing *cytokines* and *growth factors* to promote healing. As described below, however, macrophages in the arterial wall can be abnormally activated, causing a type of slow inflammatory reaction, which eventually results in advanced and clinically dangerous plaques.

Oxidized low density lipoprotein, macrophages and atherogenesis

Lipoproteins transport cholesterol and other lipids in the bloodstream (see Chapter 33). Elevated levels of one type of lipoprotein, low density lipoprotein (LDL), are associated with atherosclerosis. Native LDL is not atherogenic. However, oxidative modification of LDL by oxidants derived from macrophages and endothelial and smooth muscle cells can lead to the generation of highly atherogenic **oxidized LDL** within the vascular wall.

Oxidized LDL is thought to promote atherogenesis through several mechanisms (upper panel of Fig. 34.1). Oxidized LDL is chemotactic for (i.e. attracts) circulating monocytes, and increases the expression of endothelial cell adhesion molecules

to which monocytes attach. The monocytes then penetrate the endothelial monolayer, lodge beneath it, and mature into macrophages. Cellular uptake of native LDL is normally highly regulated. However, certain cells, including macrophages, are unable to control their uptake of oxidized LDL, which occurs via **scavenger receptors**. Once within the vascular wall, macrophages therefore accumulate large quantities of oxidized LDL, eventually becoming the cholesterol-laden **foam cells** forming the fatty streak.

As shown in the lower left of the figure, stimulation of macrophages and endothelial cells by oxidized LDL causes these cells to release cytokines. T-lymphocytes may also enter the vascular wall and release cytokines. Additional cytokines are released by platelets aggregating on the endothelium at the site at which it has been damaged by oxidized LDL and other toxic substances released by the foam cells. The cytokines act on the vascular smooth muscle cells of the media, causing them to *migrate into the intima, to proliferate,* and to *secrete abnormal amounts of collagen and other connective tissue proteins.* Over time, the intimal accumulation of smooth muscle cells and connective tissue forms the fibrous cap on the inner arterial wall. Underneath this, ongoing foam cell formation and deterioration forms a layer of extracellular lipid (largely cholesterol and cholesteryl esters) and cellular debris. Still-viable foam cells often localize at the edges or shoulders of the lesion. Underneath the lipid, the medial layer of smooth muscle cells is weakened and atrophied.

Clinical consequences of advanced atherosclerosis

Atherosclerotic lesions are of most clinical consequence when they occur in the coronary arteries. Lesions in which the fibrous cap becomes thick tend to cause a significant **stenosis**, or narrowing of the vascular lumen, which gradually comes to cause cardiac ischaemia, especially when myocardial oxygen demand rises. This leads to **stable or exertional angina** (see Chapter 37). Advanced plaques often have large areas of endothelial denudation, which serve as sites for thrombus formation. In addition, lipid- and foam-cell-rich lesions are particularly unstable and prone to tearing open. This **plaque rupture** may be favoured by the presence in the lesion of T-lymphocytes, as these produce interferon gamma which inhibits matrix formation, and of macrophages, which produce proteases that degrade the connective tissue matrix. Plaque rupture allows blood to enter the lesion, causing thrombi to form on the surface and/or within the lesion, often resulting in an acute coronary syndrome such as unstable angina (see Chapter 38) or myocardial infarction (see Chapter 41). Non-fatal chronic thrombi may gradually be replaced by connective tissue and incorporated into the lesion, a process termed **organization**. Atherosclerosis of cerebral arteries is the major cause of **stroke** (cerebral infarction). Atherosclerotic stenosis of the renal arteries causes about two-thirds of cases of **renovascular hypertension**.

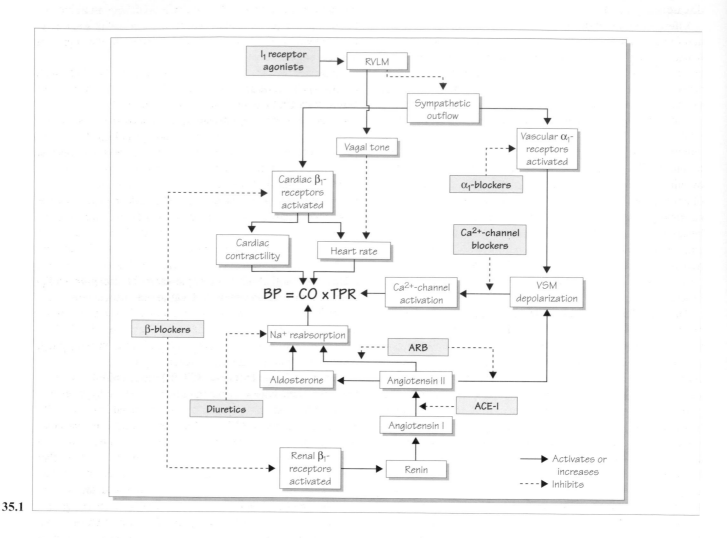

35.1

Table 35.1 Classification of adult blood pressure by the US Joint National Committee on Detection, Evaluation and Treatment of High Blood Pressure.

Classification	Systolic (mmHg)		Diastolic (mmHg)
Normotension	< 130	and/or	< 85
High normal	130–139	and/or	85–89
Stage 1 HT	140–159	and/or	90–99
Stage 2 HT	160–179	and/or	100–109
Stage 3 HT	> 180	and/or	> 110

Hypertension is defined pragmatically as the level of blood pressure above which therapeutic intervention can be shown to reduce the risk of developing cardiovascular disease (Table 35.1). Risk increases progressively with *both* systolic and diastolic blood pressure levels, and **isolated systolic hypertension** (ISH), which often develops in the elderly, is particularly de-

leterious. Individual blood pressure measurements can vary significantly, necessitating confirmation of all but severe hypertension by repeated measurements made over at least two separate occasions.

Epidemiological studies predict that a long-term 5–6-mmHg diminution of diastolic blood pressure (DBP) should reduce the incidence of stroke and CHD by about 40 and 25%, respectively. The World Health Organization recommends considering drug treatment when the DBP remains between 95 and 105 mmHg for more than 6 months, or if the DBP remains between 90 and 95 mmHg if certain risk factors are present. These include overt cardiovascular disease, diabetes, obesity, dyslipidaemia, a family history of cardiovascular disease, or disease of target organs vulnerable to hypertension (e.g. kidneys and brain). There is an emerging consensus that mild hypertension should be treated if a patient's overall risk of cardiovascular events (e.g. MI), as estimated using risk tables derived from the Framingham study (see Chapter 31), exceeds 2% per year. The goal of antihypertensive therapy is to reduce the blood pressure to below 140/90 mmHg (or to below 135/85 in diabetics and those with renal disease).

Lifestyle modifications such as *weight reduction, regular aerobic exercise* and *limitation of dietary sodium* and *alcohol intake* can often normalize pressure in mild hypertensives. They are also useful adjuncts to pharmacological therapy of more severe disease, and have the important added bonus of reducing overall cardiovascular risk.

Antihypertensive drugs act to reduce cardiac output and/or total peripheral resistance. Of the various classes available, diuretics or β-blockers are usually recommended as initial drugs for uncomplicated hypertension because these have been shown by clinical trials to reduce mortality. However, as other types of antihypertensive drugs can often exert beneficial actions on coexisting conditions (e.g. ACE inhibitors in heart failure, diabetes), these drugs may be more appropriate for some patients. Inadequate or adverse responses to the first drug tried necessitate substitution with an agent from another class. In the majority of cases, combinations of two or three drugs are needed to achieve adequate blood pressure control.

Thiazide diuretics cause an initial increased Na^+ excretion by the kidneys, which is due to inhibition of Na^+/Cl^- symport in the distal nephron. This leads to a fall in blood volume and cardiac output. Subsequently, blood volume recovers, but total peripheral resistance falls due to an unknown mechanism (possibly the opening of ATP-dependent K^+ channels in vascular smooth muscle cells). Diuretics can be combined with vasodilators (e.g. α_1-blockers, Ca^{2+}-channel antagonists), which may elicit volume expansion and oedema due to renin–angiotensin–aldosterone system activation. Diuretics cause hypokalaemia by promoting Na^+/K^+ exchange in the collecting tubule (see Chapter 45). This can be prevented by also giving K^+-sparing diuretics (e.g. amiloride) to reduce Na^+ reabsorption by blocking Na^+ channels in the collecting duct. Additional side effects can include increases in plasma insulin, glucose or cholesterol, as well as hypersensitivity reactions and impotence. In the 2002 ALLHAT study, the diuretic chlorthalidone lowered blood pressure as well as amlodipine and lisinopril (see below), and was superior to both at preventing major cardiovascular disease.

β-receptor blockers antagonize sympathetic nervous system stimulation of cardiac β-receptors (mainly β_1), thereby reducing cardiac output via negative inotropic and chronotropic effects. They also block β-receptors on juxtaglomerular granule cells in the kidney, thus inhibiting renin release and reducing plasma levels of angiotensin II and aldosterone. During treatment, total peripheral resistance rises initially and then returns to the pre-drug level via an unknown mechanism, while cardiac output remains depressed. Some β-blockers are selective for the β_1 subtype (atenolol), while others block both β_1 and β_2 subtypes (propranolol), and several (pindolol) are partial β-receptor agonists. In each case, the effects on blood pressure are similar, although the partial β-receptor agonists are probably acting more as

vasodilators than by reducing cardiac output. All β-blockers are contraindicated in asthma due to their potential effects on bronchiolar β_2-receptors. Adverse effects of these drugs include fatigue, negative inotropy, CNS disturbances with some (e.g. nightmares), and worsening and masking of the signs of hypoglycaemia.

Angiotensin-converting enzyme inhibitors (ACE-I) such as **captopril**, **enalopril** and **lisinopril** block the conversion of angiotensin I into angiotensin II. This reduces total peripheral resistance because angiotensin II stimulates the sympathetic system centrally, promotes release of norepinephrine from sympathetic nerves, and vasoconstricts directly. The fall in plasma angiotensin, and consequently in aldosterone, also promotes diuresis/natriuresis, because both hormones cause renal Na^+ and water retention (see Chapter 28). ACE also metabolizes the vasodilator bradykinin, and part of the beneficial action of ACE-I may be due to elevated levels of bradykinin. Increases in bradykinin may also, however, be responsible for the chronic cough which is the most common adverse effect of ACE-I. This effect does not occur with **angiotensin II receptor (AT_1) blockers** such as **losartan** and **valsartan**, which selectively inhibit the effects of angiotensin II on its AT_1 subtype without affecting bradykinin levels. Both ACE-I and the AT_1 blockers have few side effects, but are contraindicated in pregnancy, renovascular disease and aortic stenosis.

Calcium-channel blockers (CCBs) such as **nifedipine**, **verapamil** and **diltiazem** are commonly used to treat hypertension due to their vasodilating properties, as described in Chapter 39. The dihydropyridine CCBs, which are selective for vascular smooth muscle over the heart, are used most widely, and also have a useful diuretic effect. Recent clinical trials show that the longer acting dihydropyridine CCBs such as nitrendipine and felodipine are comparable to β-blockers and diuretics in reducing morbidity and mortality, especially in certain groups such as the elderly. Rapidly acting dihydropyridine CCBs are no longer recommended since they may increase mortality via pro-ischaemic and other effects.

α_1-receptor-selective blockers are second-line antihypertensives, which cause vasodilatation by inhibiting the ongoing constriction of arteries by the sympathetic neurotransmitter norepinephrine. These drugs are used in preference to non-selective α-antagonists in order to prevent the increased norepinephrine release from sympathetic nerves, which would occur if presynaptic α_2-receptors were also blocked. The relatively new drugs **rilmenidine** and **moxonidine** reduce sympathetic outflow by activating central *imidazoline* (I_1) receptors in the rostral ventrolateral medulla (RVLM). This lowers blood pressure with few side effects, but the use of these drugs is limited due to the present lack of evidence from clinical trials that these drugs have beneficial effects on survival.

In cases in which hypertension is secondary to a known condition or factor (e.g. renal stenosis, oral contraceptives), removal of this cause is often sufficient to normalize the blood pressure.

36 Mechanisms of primary hypertension

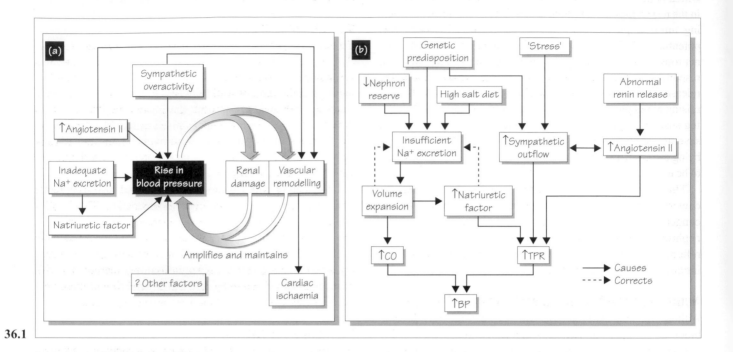

36.1

In > 90% of cases, hypertension has no obvious cause, and is termed **primary** or **essential**. Primary hypertension is a **multifactorial genetic disorder**, in which inheritance of a number of abnormal genes predisposes an individual to high blood pressure, especially if appropriate *environmental influences* (e.g. high salt diet, psychosocial stress) are also present. The identities of the genes involved are presently unresolved. Attempts to define causative mechanisms have mainly focused on uncovering functional abnormalities associated with hypertension. Many such studies have been carried out in strains of animals which have been selectively bred to develop high blood pressure, in the hope that the mechanisms causing hypertension are similar across species.

Studies tracking cardiovascular function over many years have shown that early human hypertension is often associated with an increased cardiac output (CO) and heart rate, but a normal total peripheral resistance (TPR). Over a period of years, CO falls to subnormal levels, while TPR becomes permanently increased, thereby maintaining the hypertension (recall that blood pressure = CO × TPR). One important implication of these observations is that the factors maintaining high blood pressure may change over time. Therefore the mechanisms which initiate high blood pressure (e.g. insufficient Na+ excretion, sympathetic overactivity), may then be succeeded and/or amplified by additional common secondary mechanisms (e.g. renal damage and vascular structural remodelling) which are caused by, and maintain, the initial rise in pressure. This unifying hypothesis for primary hypertension is shown in Fig. 36.1(a).

The kidney and sodium in hypertension

The pressure–natriuresis model: The kidneys regulate long-term blood pressure by controlling the body's Na+ content (see Chapter 28). Guyton has proposed that hypertension is caused by renal abnormalities which cause *impaired* or *inadequate Na+ excretion* (Fig. 36.1b). According to this model, the resulting Na+ retention increases blood volume, and therefore CO and blood pressure. These changes then promote Na+ excretion by causing pressure natriuresis (see Chapter 28). Fluid balance is therefore restored, but at the cost of a rise in blood pressure. Over the long term, the rise in blood pressure or flow would set in train *auto-regulatory* processes resulting in vasoconstriction and/or vascular structural remodelling. This would reduce blood volume to normal levels, but by raising TPR would maintain the high blood pressure needed for Na+ balance.

There is extensive evidence that a renal mechanism of hypertension is important in many people. For example, a high salt diet, which should exacerbate the renal deficiency in Na+ excretion, worsens hypertension in many patients and, as shown in the Intersalt study, seems to cause a slow rise in blood pressure over many years in most people. It has also been shown that blood pressure falls when the kidneys from normotensives are transplanted into hypertensives. Impairment of renal Na+ excretion has been demonstrated directly in the *Liddle syndrome*, a rare form of hypertension in which a mutation of the mineralocorticoid-sensitive Na+ channel causes its continual overactivity.

The natriuretic factor hypothesis: de Wardener and others have proposed that the body responds to inadequate renal salt excretion by producing one or more **natriuretic factors** (not to be confused with **atrial natriuretic peptide**, see Chapter 28) which promote salt excretion by inhibiting the Na^+,K^+-ATPase in the nephron. Na^+ pumps are also indirectly involved in lowering intracellular Ca^{2+}, via regulation of both the membrane potential and Na^+–Ca^{2+} exchange in smooth muscle cells and neurons. Natriuretic factors would therefore cause additional responses such as vasoconstriction, increased norepinephrine release, and possibly stimulation of brain centres involved in raising blood pressure. These effects would increase TPR, causing sustained hypertension. In agreement with this hypothesis, several endogenous substances that inhibit the Na^+ pump, one being almost identical in structure to ouabain, have been found to be elevated in the plasma from hypertensives.

The reduced nephron number hypothesis: Brenner and coworkers have proposed that many hypertensives have a congenital reduction in the number, or filtering ability, of their nephrons which would cause the inadequate Na^+ excretion referred to above. Evidence suggests that this may arise from intrauterine growth retardation.

Neurogenic and humoral theories of hypertension

Although renin release should be greatly suppressed by elevated blood pressure, many hypertensives have normal or even high plasma renin activity. Laragh and coworkers have proposed that many hypertensives have an *abnormality of renin release* which would lead both to increased angiotensin II-mediated vasoconstriction and to Na^+ retention via aldosterone, both mechanisms causing hypertension. Angiotensin II is also a potent stimulator of the sympathetic nervous system. Primary hypertension in some individuals has also been linked to a mutation in the **angiotensinogen** gene, which could promote increased angiotensin II production.

The **neurogenic model of hypertension** suggests that blood pressure elevation is primarily initiated by defective neurohumoral regulation of blood pressure. Supporters of this concept stress that the central nervous system is ultimately the final determinant of blood pressure, because it can exert long-term influences on renal function (e.g. renal bloodflow), on the production of vasoactive substances, and on vascular and cardiac structure. The neurogenic model is supported by evidence that sympathetic nervous activity is increased in young borderline hypertensives, and also by the fact that drugs which reduce sympathetic outflow effectively lower blood pressure (see Chapter 35). It may also explain studies in which psychosocial stress has been linked to hypertension.

Insulin resistance is a condition in which the body becomes less responsive to the actions of the hormone *insulin*, leading to a compensatory rise in plasma insulin levels. Both insulin resistance and obesity, with which it is often associated, are very common in hypertensives. There is evidence that excessive insulin can cause multiple effects on the body which could promote hypertension, including activation of the sympathetic nervous system, increased renal Na^+ reabsorption, and reduced endothelium-dependent vasodilatation.

Vascular remodelling

Established hypertension is associated with the *structural alteration* of small arteries and larger arterioles. This process, termed **remodelling**, results in the narrowing of these vessels and an increase in the ratio of wall thickness to luminal radius. These changes are thought to constitute an adaptive mechanism which protects the microcirculation from increased blood pressure. Remodelling may also be enhanced by the renin–angiotensin–aldosterone and sympathetic nervous systems, the activation of which are known to promote smooth muscle cell growth.

Remodelling will increase basal TPR and also exaggerate any increase in TPR caused by vasoconstriction. This implies that remodelling would accentuate increases in blood pressure caused by other factors, thereby contributing to the vicious cycle illustrated in Fig. 36.1(a). In addition, remodelling of the coronary arteries as a result of hypertension may increase the risk of myocardial infarction by restricting the ability of these vessels to increase the cardiac blood supply during ischaemia.

Secondary hypertension

In < 10% of cases, high blood pressure is secondary to a known condition or factor. Common causes of **secondary hypertension** include:

1 *Renal parenchymal* and *renovascular diseases*, which impair volume regulation and/or activate the renin–angiotensin–aldosterone system.
2 *Endocrine disturbances*, often of the adrenal cortex, and associated with oversecretion of aldosterone, cortisol and/or catecholamines.
3 *Oral contraceptives*, which may raise blood pressure via renin–angiotensin–aldosterone activation and hyperinsulinaemia.

Malignant or accelerated hypertension is an uncommon condition which develops quickly, involves large elevations in pressure, is often secondary to other conditions, rapidly damages the kidneys, retina, brain and heart, and if untreated causes death within 1–2 years.

Consequences of hypertension

Chronic hypertension causes changes in the arteries similar to those due to ageing. These include endothelial damage and **arteriosclerosis**, a thickening and increased connective tissue content of the arterial wall that reduces arterial compliance. These effects on vascular structure combine with elevated arterial pressure to promote atherosclerosis, coronary heart disease, left ventricular hypertrophy and renal damage. Hypertension is therefore an important risk factor for *myocardial infarction*, *congestive heart failure*, *stroke* and *renal failure*.

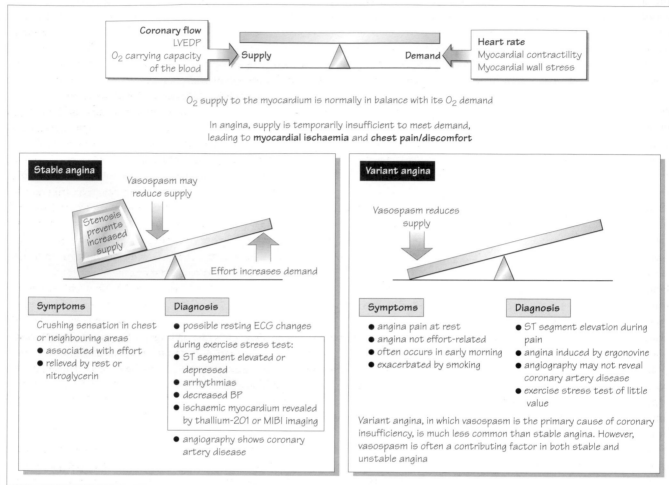

Angina pectoris is an episodic pain or crushing/squeezing sensation in the chest caused by reversible myocardial ischaemia. The discomfort may radiate into the neck, jaw and arms (particularly the left) and, more rarely, into the back. Other common symptoms include shortness of breath, abdominal pain and dizziness. Syncope (collapse) occurs infrequently. Ischaemia may produce classic angina or may be totally *silent* without any symptoms. The clinical outlook from silent ischaemia is similar to symptomatic angina.

Three forms of angina are recognized. **Stable** and **variant** angina are discussed below, and **unstable angina** is described in Chapter 38.

Pathophysiology

Figure 37.1 shows the factors that determine myocardial O_2 supply and demand. O_2 demand is determined by **heart rate**, **left ventricular contractility** and **systolic wall stress**, and therefore increases with **exercise**, **hypertension** and **left ventricular**

dilatation (e.g. during chronic heart failure). Myocardial O_2 supply is primarily determined by coronary bloodflow and coronary vascular resistance, which mostly occurs at the level of the intramyocardial arterioles. With exercise the coronary bloodflow can increase to four to six times baseline, which is the normal coronary flow reserve (see Chapter 24).

Stable or **exertional/typical** angina arises when the flow reserve of one or more coronary arteries is limited by a significant structural stenosis (> 70%) resulting from atherosclerotic coronary heart disease. Stenoses typically develop in the epicardial region of arteries, within 6 cm of the aorta. Under resting conditions, cardiac O_2 demand is low enough to be satisfied even by a diminished coronary flow. When, however, exertion or emotional stress increases myocardial O_2 demand, dilatation of the nondiseased areas of the artery is unable to increase the supply of blood to the heart because stenosis presents a fixed, nondilating obstruction. The resulting imbalance between myocardial O_2 demand and supply causes myocardial ischaemia.

Ischaemia develops mainly in the **subendocardium**, the inner part of the myocardial wall. As described in Chapter 24, the bloodflow to the left ventricular wall occurs mainly during diastole, as a result of arteriolar compression during systole. The arterioles of the subendocardium are compressed more than those of the mid- or subepicardial layers, so that the subendocardium is most vulnerable to a relative lack of O_2.

In addition to causing pain, ischaemia causes a decline in myocardial cell high-energy phosphates (creatine phosphate and ATP). As a result, both ventricular contractility and diastolic relaxation in the territory of affected arteries are impaired. Consequences of these events may include a fall in cardiac output, symptoms of pulmonary congestion, and activation of the sympathetic nervous system. Stable angina is almost always relieved within 5–10 min by rest or by nitroglycerin, which reduces cardiac O_2 demand.

Some patients with stable angina may have excellent effort tolerance one day, but develop angina with minimal activity on another day. Contributing to this phenomenon of *variable threshold angina* is a dynamic endothelial dysfunction that often occurs in patients with coronary artery disease. The endothelium normally acts via nitric oxide to dilate coronary arteries during exercise. If this endothelium-dependent vasodilatation is periodically impaired, exercise may result in paradoxical vasoconstriction as a result of the unopposed vasoconstricting effect of the sympathetic nervous system on coronary α-receptors.

Variant angina, also termed **vasospastic** or **Prinzmetal's** angina, is an uncommon condition in which myocardial ischaemia and pain are caused by a severe transient *occlusive spasm* of one or more epicardial coronary arteries. Patients with variant angina may or may not have coronary atherosclerotosis, and in the former case, vasospasm ofter occurs in the vicinity of plaques. Variant angina occurs at rest (typically in the early morning hours) and may be intensely painful. It is exacerbated by smoking, and can be precipitated by cocaine use. About 30% of these patients show no evidence of coronary atherosclerotic lesions. Vasospasm is thought to occur because a segment of artery becomes abnormally over-reactive to vasoconstricting agents (e.g. norepinephrine, serotonin). There is also evidence that flow-mediated vasodilatation, a function of the endothelium, is impaired in the coronary arteries of patients with variant angina, and that this endothelial dysfunction may be due to oxidative stress (see Chapter 23).

Diagnosis

Ischaemic heart disease and stable angina can be distinguished from other conditions causing chest pain (e.g. neuromuscular disorders, gastroesophageal reflux) on the basis of characteristic anginal symptoms and several types of diagnostic investigation. Although *resting ST/T wave changes* indicate severe underlying coronary artery disease, the resting ECG is often normal. In this case, the presence of ischaemic heart disease can be unmasked by an **exercise stress test**, during which patients exercise at a progressively increasing level of effort on a stationary bicycle or treadmill. Development of cardiac ischaemia is revealed by chest pain, ECG changes including *ST segment depression* or *elevation*, arrhythmias, or a fall in blood pressure due to reduced ventricular contractility. The degree of effort at which these signs develop indicates the severity of ischaemia.

The exercise stress test is less useful in uncovering ischaemia-related ECG changes if the baseline ECG is already abnormal as a result of factors such as left bundle branch block. In such patients, techniques designed to visualize ischaemic myocardium can be combined with the stress test to increase its specificity. **Thallium-201** is an isotope that is taken up by normal but not ischaemic or previously infarcted myocardium. It is given intravenously during the stress test, and a gamma camera is used to image its distribution in the heart both immediately and also after the test, when ischaemia has subsided. A region of exercise-induced ischaemia will cause a 'cold spot' during but not after the stress test, because it will take up thallium-201 only when ischaemia has passed. **99mTc-methoxy isobutyl isonitrile** (MIBI) can also be used for this purpose. **Coronary angiography** (see Chapter 32) is used to provide direct radiographic visualization of the extent and severity of coronary artery disease, allowing risk assessment.

The hallmark of variant angina is ST segment elevation on the ECG. Cardiac ischaemia caused by variant angina may cause ventricular arrhythmias, syncope (unconsciousness) and even myocardial infarction during prolonged attacks. Variant angina can be provoked by intravenous administration of the vasoconstrictor **ergonovine**, forming the basis of a hospital test for this condition.

Prognosis
Stable angina
Mortality is 2–4% a year if only one coronary artery is diseased, but increases with the number of diseased arteries, especially if there is significant stenosis in the left coronary artery mainstem. Patients with poor left ventricular function are at particular risk.

Variant angina
Patients without significant coronary artery disease have a benign prognosis; in a recent study only 4% of patients in this group died from a cardiac cause during an average follow-up period of 7 years. However, patients who also have severe coronary artery disease or who develop severe arrhythmias during vasospastic episodes are at greater risk.

Management
The management of angina is designed to control symptoms, reduce underlying risk factors, and improve prognosis. **Control of symptoms** involves the use of nitrovasodilators, β-adrenoceptor blockers and Ca^{2+}-channel antagonists (see Chapter 39). Minimization of **risk factors** involves the use of low-dose aspirin, lipid-lowering drugs and lifestyle changes, and is a vital component of treatment. Stable angina can also be treated using the **revascularization** techniques described in Chapter 40.

38 Unstable angina and non-ST segment elevation myocardial infarction

38.1

Stable angina is a chronic condition which occurs on a relatively predictable basis when cardiac ischaemia develops due to the inability of a narrowed coronary artery to meet an increased cardiac oxygen demand. Conversely, the **acute coronary syndromes (ACS)**, including in ascending order of severity, **unstable angina**, **non-ST segment elevation myocardial infarction (NSTEMI)** and **ST elevation myocardial infarction (STEMI)**, represent a spectrum of dangerous conditions in which myocardial ischaemia results from *a sudden decrease in the flow of blood through a coronary vessel*. This decrease is almost always initiated by the rupture of an atherosclerotic plaque, resulting in the formation of an intracoronary thrombus which diminishes or abolishes the flow of blood.

When a patient presents with a suspected acute coronary syndrome, an ECG is immediately carried out (see Fig. 38.1 upper left). The hallmark of **STEMI**, the most serious acute coronary syndrome, is *sustained elevation of the ST segment of the ECG*. This indicates that a large area of the myocardium, probably involving the full thickness of a ventricular wall, has suffered *necrosis* (cell death, with subsequent inflammation and scarring) as a result of prolonged ischaemia. Myocardial necrosis causes the release of intracellular proteins, such as **troponins T and I**. These can be detected in the blood, and act as markers of

myocardial cell death. STEMI is confirmed when elevated levels of these markers are found. STEMI typically occurs when a thrombus has completely occluded a coronary artery for a significant amount of time, and usually causes more severe symptoms than do unstable angina or NSTEMI.

Incomplete or temporary coronary occlusion, or the existence of collateral coronary arteries which can maintain some supply of blood to the affected region, may result in a smaller degree of myocardial ischaemia and necrosis, usually limited to the subendocardium. This may not result in ST segment elevation, but does cause the release of markers of necrosis. Patients who are found to have elevated levels of these markers, but who do not have ST segment elevation, are deemed to have suffered **NSTEMI**.

Patients who demonstrate symptoms associated with ACS, but who have neither ST segment elevation nor elevated levels of markers of myocardial necrosis, are deemed to have **unstable angina (UA)**. In this case, it is likely that the coronary obstruction has been of limited extent and/or duration (< 20 min), and is thus sufficient to cause ischaemia but not detectable necrosis.

Both NSTEMI and STEMI are grouped together as **acute myocardial infarctions**, but are managed differently, in that pharmacological reperfusion (thrombolysis) is used to treat STEMI but not NSTEMI (see Chapters 41, 42). On the other hand, the management of unstable angina and NSTEMI utilizes overlapping approaches, and these conditions are often discussed together as 'UA/NSTEMI'. Symptoms of UA/NSTEMI resemble those of stable angina, but they are frequently more painful, intense and persistent, often lasting 30 min. Pain is frequently resistant to nitroglycerin. Typical patient presentations include:

1 Crescendo angina, where attacks are progressively more severe, prolonged and frequent.

2 Angina of recent onset brought on by minimal exertion.

3 Angina at rest/with minimal exertion or during sleep.

4 Post-MI angina (ischaemic pain 24 h to 2 weeks after MI).

Pathophysiology of UA/NSTEMI

Studies have shown that episodes of unstable angina are preceded by a fall in coronary bloodflow, thought to result from the periodic development of coronary **thrombosis** and **vasoconstriction**, which are triggered by coronary artery disease (Fig. 38.1).

Thrombosis is promoted by the endothelial damage and turbulent bloodflow associated with atherosclerotic plaques. Compared to the lesions of stable angina, plaques found in patients with acute coronary syndromes tend to have a thinner fibrous cap and a larger lipid core, and are generally more widespread and severe. These stenoses are often *eccentric*—the plaque does not surround the entire circumference of the artery. Such lesions are especially vulnerable to being ruptured by haemodynamic stress. This exposes the plaque interior, which powerfully stimulates platelet aggregation and thrombosis. The thrombus propagates out into the coronary lumen, occluding the artery. Rupture may also cause haemorrhage into the lesion itself, expanding it out into the lumen and worsening stenosis.

These events may be exacerbated by impaired coronary vasodilatation, and vasospasm due to plaque-associated endothelial damage, which reduces the local release of endothelium-dependent relaxing factors. Platelet aggregation and thrombosis also cause the local generation of vasoconstrictors such as thromboxane A_2 and serotonin.

Risk stratification

The occurrence of UA and NSTEMI indicates that a patient has a high risk of undergoing subsequent episodes of coronary thrombosis which may cause more significant cardiac damage or death. In the USA, for example, ~4% of the 1.3 million people who enter hospital with UA/NSTEMI die within 30 days, and ~8% suffer (re)infarction. Although NSTEMI is by definition a more serious 'event' than is UA, these are both heterogeneous conditions, and the risk of suffering (re)infarction is higher in some patients with UA than in others with NSTEMI. Risk assessment is therefore of paramount importance. Risk is scored on the basis of a number of factors, including frequency and severity of angina, elevated markers of cardiac necrosis, ECG changes (ST segment depression and/or T-wave inversion), and

prior angiographic evidence of atherosclerotic plaque (see also Chapter 52).

Management

UA/NSTEMI is a medical emergency. Typically, treatment begins with aggressive pharmacological therapy, which focuses on rendering the acute coronary lesion less dangerous, minimizing residual ischaemia, and preventing future coronary events. **Urgent revascularization** is considered for patients with high-risk and/or very significant coronary artery disease, or if drug treatment fails to control symptoms (Chapter 40).

Drug treatment of UA/NSTEMI (see also Chapter 43 for drug mechanisms)

Antiplatelet therapy: All patients with UA/NSTEMI are immediately treated with **low-dose aspirin**, which is then continued indefinitely, in order to suppress platelet aggregation, a key initial step in thrombosis. Clinical trials have shown that aspirin, in doses as low as 75 mg/day, reduces mortality or infarction in this group by more than 50%.

The thienopyridine **clopidogrel**, which inhibits ADP-stimulated platelet aggregation, was shown in the 2000 CURE trial to reduce cardiovascular morbidity and mortality by ~20% in patients with UA/NSTEMI. It is recommended that clopidogrel should be added in with aspirin therapy for at least a month, although the optimal duration of its use is not yet defined.

Glycoprotein IIb/IIIa antagonists are the most powerful of the antiplatelet drugs. These drugs are of proven benefit in UA/NSTEMI patients who receive percutaneous transcoronary angioplasty (PCTA), a type of revascularization procedure in which plaque-stenosed coronary arteries are widened using a balloon catheter (see Chapter 40). PCTA usually involves placing a stent (a mesh tube) in the affected coronary to keep it open, and the glycoprotein IIb/IIIa antagonists reduce the tendency of stents to cause thrombosis.

Anticoagulant therapy: Unfractionated heparin (UH) or **low molecular weight heparins (LMWH)**, which inhibit the coagulation cascade mainly at factor X and thrombin, are given to all patients with UA/NSTEMI. These drugs are given intravenously (UH) or subcutaneously (LMWH) while patients are hospitalized, but not routinely thereafter. There is evidence that the LMWH enoxaparin may be preferable to UH.

Other drugs: β-blockers have been shown to reduce cardiovascular morbidity and mortality in patients with UA/NSTEMI, and should be given unless contraindicated (e.g. in asthma). **Nitrates** can be given, especially on a temporary basis, to relieve pain, but do not appear to affect mortality. **Ca²⁺-channel blockers** should *not* be used to treat UA/NSTEMI, although they may be continued if the patient is already receiving them for chronic stable angina. On the other hand, there is increasing evidence that the lipid-lowering '**statins**' and **angiotensin-converting enzyme inhibitors** improve survival in UA/NSTEMI.

39 Pharmacological management of stable and variant angina

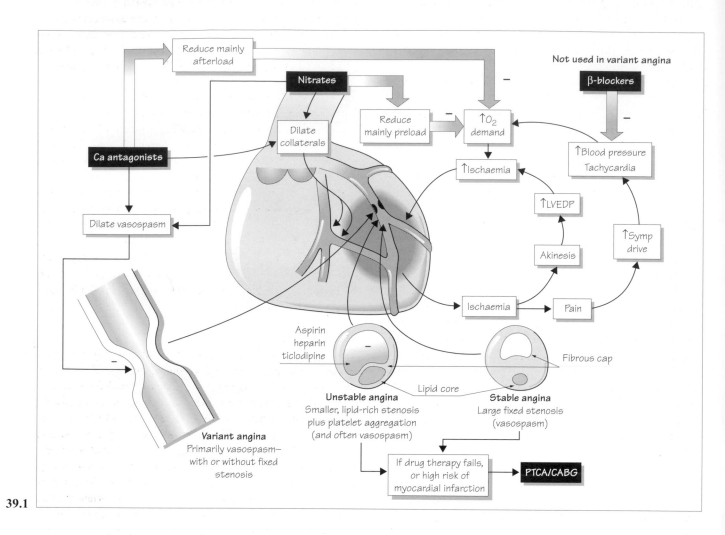

39.1

Treatment of chronic angina is designed both to control symptoms, and also to prevent the progression of coronary heart disease by reducing relevant risk factors. Angina symptoms are controlled by restoring the balance between myocardial O_2 demand and supply. In **stable angina**, the bloodflow through stenotic coronary arteries is limited, and therapy is mainly aimed at reducing O_2 demand with **vasodilators** and **β-blockers**. The treatment of **variant angina** is primarily directed at reversing coronary **vasospasm**.

Nitrovasodilators

Nitrovasodilators include **nitroglycerin** (glyceryl trinitrate), **isosorbide mononitrate**, **isosorbide dinitrate**, **erythrityl tetranitrate** and **pentaerythritol tetranitrate**. Rapidly acting nitrovasodilators are used to prevent angina, or to terminate ongoing attacks, while longer acting preparations are combined with other drugs to provide long-term prophylaxis.

Nitrovasodilators act as a 'pharmacological endothelium'.

They react with cellular thiols (-SH groups) in vascular smooth muscle cells, thereby releasing nitrite ions (NO_2^-). These are then reduced to nitric oxide, which stimulates guanylate cyclase to elevate cGMP, thereby causing vasodilatation (see Chapter 23). At therapeutic doses, nitrovasodilators act primarily to dilate veins, thus reducing central venous pressure (preload) and ventricular end-diastolic volume. This lowers myocardial contraction, wall stress and O_2 demand. Some arterial dilatation also occurs, diminishing total peripheral resistance (afterload). This allows the left ventricle to maintain cardiac output with a smaller stroke volume, again decreasing O_2 demand.

Nitrovasodilators can also increase the perfusion of ischaemic myocardium by several mechanisms. They dilate coronary **collateral vessels** (see Chapter 3). These often increase in number and diameter in the presence of a significant stenosis, providing alternative perfusion of ischaemic zones. Nitrovasodilators also relieve coronary vasospasm, and help to diminish plaque-related platelet aggregation and thrombosis by elevating platelet cGMP.

Nitroglycerin and isosorbide dinitrate taken sublingually relieve angina within minutes; this route of administration avoids the extensive first-pass metabolism of these drugs associated with oral dosing. These and other nitrovasodilators can also be given in slowly absorbed oral, transdermal and buccal forms for sustained effect.

Continuous exposure to nitrovasodilators causes **tolerance**, which may in part be caused by the depletion of tissue thiols. Tolerance is irrelevant with short-acting nitrovasodilators, but long-acting preparations become ineffective within hours. Tolerance can be minimized by 'eccentric' dosing schedules that allow blood concentrations to become low overnight. The most important adverse effect of nitrovasodilators is headache. Reflex tachycardia and orthostatic hypotension may also occur.

Ca^{2+}-channel blockers (CCBs; also Ca^{2+} antagonists)

These drugs act by blocking the voltage-gated Ca^{2+} channels that allow depolarization-mediated influx of Ca^{2+} into smooth muscle cells, and also cardiac myocytes (see Chapters 11, 12). The interaction of blocker and Ca^{2+} channel is best understood for the *dihydropyridines*, which include **nifedipine**, **amlodipine** and **felodipine**. The affinity of dihydropyridines for the channel increases enormously when the channel is in its *inactivated* state (see Chapter 10). Channel inactivation is favoured by a less negative membrane potential (Em). Dihydropyridines therefore have a relatively selective effect on vascular muscle (Em ~–50) compared to cardiac muscle (Em ~–80). This selectivity is further enhanced because dihydropyridine-mediated vasodilatation stimulates the baroreceptor reflex, overcoming any direct negative inotropic effects.

The phenylalkylamine **verapamil** interacts preferentially with the channel in its *open* state. Verapamil binding is therefore less dependent on membrane potential; and both cardiac and vascular Ca^{2+} channels are blocked. Verapamil therefore has negative inotropic effects and severely depresses AV nodal conduction. The benzothiazepine **diltiazem** has intermediate properties; at therapeutic doses it vasodilates but also depresses AV conduction and has negative inotropic/chronotropic effects.

CCBs prevent angina mainly by causing arteriolar vasodilatation and decreasing afterload. They also prevent coronary vasospasm, making them particularly useful in variant angina. Their use is theoretically advantageous in variable threshold angina, in which coronary vasoconstriction is thought to contribute to reduced cardiac perfusion (see Chapter 37). The negative inotropic and chronotropic effects of verapamil and diltiazem also contribute to their usefulness by reducing myocardial O$_2$ demand.

The vasodilatation caused by CCBs can cause hypotension, headache and peripheral oedema (mainly dihydropyridines). On the other hand, their cardiac effects can elicit excessive cardiodepression and AV node conduction block (mainly verapamil and diltiazem). These drugs are contraindicated in heart failure, especially if β-blockers are being used.

β-Adrenergic receptor blockers

As Fig. 39.1 illustrates, myocardial ischaemia creates a vicious cycle by activating the sympathetic system and increasing ventricular end-diastolic pressure; both these effects then worsen ischaemia and anginal pain. **β-blockers**, which are used for the prophylaxis of angina, help to block this cycle, thereby decreasing O$_2$ demand. They further reduce O$_2$ demand by decreasing myocardial contractility and wall stress. The resting and exercising heart rate also falls. This increases the fraction of time the heart spends in diastole, thus enhancing perfusion of the left ventricle, which occurs predominantly during diastole. The main therapeutic action of these drugs is on cardiac β$_1$-receptors, but both β$_1$-selective and (β$_1$/β$_2$) nonselective blockers are used.

β-blockers can have a variety of adverse effects, including fatigue, reduced left ventricular function and severe bradycardia. They can precipitate asthma by blocking β$_2$-receptors in the airways, and therefore even β$_1$-selective agents are contraindicated in this condition. Lipid-soluble β-blockers (e.g. propranolol) can enter the central nervous system and cause depression or nightmares. β-blockers can also worsen insulin-induced hypoglycaemia in diabetics.

Management of angina

Therapy is typically instituted with a short-acting nitrovasodilator taken to prevent and terminate attacks. If control is insufficient, a Ca^{2+} antagonist or β-blocker is added for prophylaxis. The choice between these is influenced by coexisting conditions and contraindications. For example, a CCB is preferable if the patient also suffers from asthma or hypertension, and a β-blocker may be superior if atrial fibrillation is also present. If needed, this regimen can be supplemented with a long-acting nitrovasodilator. Finally, a combination of all of these agents can be employed. β-blockers are *not* used in variant angina, as they may worsen coronary vasospasm by blocking the β$_2$- (vasodilating), but not α$_1$- (vasoconstricting) mediated effects of sympathetic stimulation. If angina symptoms are refractory to drug treatment, or if the patient is at risk from widespread and serious coronary atherosclerosis, **revascularization** (see Chapter 40) is likely to be a preferred option.

Reduction of coronary risk factors

The reduction of risk factors that can contribute to the further progression of coronary heart disease has become a key focus of angina management. Angina patients should be treated with daily low-dose aspirin, which suppresses platelet aggregation and greatly reduces the risk of myocardial infarction and death in patients with both stable and unstable angina. Many are now also treated with 'statins' (see Chapter 33) to reduce their plasma LDL levels to below 100 mg/dl (2.6 mmol/L). The 2001 HOPE trial showed that the angiotensin-converting enzyme inhibitor (ACE-I) ramipril reduced the progression of atherosclerosis and enhanced survival over a period of 5 years, in a group with coronary artery disease or diabetes, suggesting that ACE-I should also considered in those with stable angina.

40 Revascularization

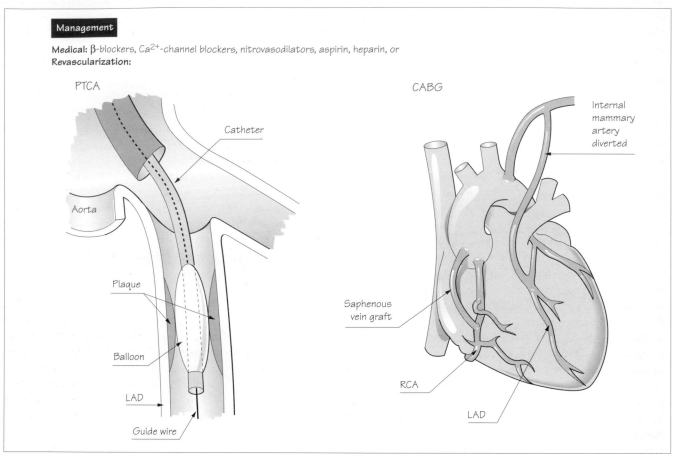

PTCA

Catheter

Aorta

Plaque

Balloon

LAD

Guide wire

CABG

Internal mammary artery diverted

Saphenous vein graft

RCA

LAD

40.1

Coronary artery bypass grafting (CABG) and **percutaneous transcoronary angioplasty (PTCA)** are revascularization techniques that are used to treat patients with both stable angina and acute coronary syndromes. As described below, both procedures are used in higher risk patients, with the choice of which technique to use determined by several factors including severity of disease and the wishes of the individual. In 1999, the last year for which full data are available, there were over 1 million coronary angioplasties, and approximately half that many CABG procedures, performed in the USA.

CABG is a surgical procedure (Fig. 40.1, right) that was first performed in 1964. Lengths of healthy superfluous blood vessels (conduits) are attached between the aorta and the coronary arteries distal to any stenosis. This allows a supply of blood to the heart, which bypasses the stenosis. Conduits commonly used for CABG include **saphenous vein** segments harvested from the leg. These, however, have limited long-term patency due to early postoperative thrombosis, intimal hyperplasia with smooth muscle proliferation in the first year, and the development of atherosclerosis after approximately 5–7 years. For this reason, the **left internal mammary artery (LIMA)** is co...

for grafting much more widely than the saphenous vein. In most cases, the LIMA is not disconnected from its parent (subclavian) artery, but is cut distally and attached to the coronary artery. Unlike the saphenous vein, the LIMA rarely becomes atherosclerotic after grafting. Patients with a LIMA graft to the crucial left anterior descending coronary artery have improved long-term survival compared to patients receiving saphenous vein grafts. The right internal mammary, gastroepiploic and radial arteries can also be used for grafting.

CABG is usually done with the patient on cardiopulmonary bypass, with the heart stopped. Blood is typically removed from the right atrium, drained into a reservoir, and then pumped through an oxygenator, then a filter and back into the aorta to perfuse the systemic circulation. The main complications of the procedure are atrial fibrillation and persistent neurological abnormalities. These latter are thought to be caused by emboli, either formed in the bypass circuit or produced by disturbance of aortic plaques during cannulation, which lodge in the cerebral vasculature. The mortality rate associated with CABG is ~2%.

PTCA, first used in 1977, is a much less invasive procedure. ...theter is introduced via the femoral, brachial or radial artery, and is positioned near the target stenosis. A guiding wire is then advanced down the lumen of the coronary artery until it is positioned across the stenosis. A balloon catheter is advanced over this wire, and then inflated at the site of the stenosis to increase the luminal diameter (Fig. 40.1, left). Emergency CABG is required in 1–2% of patients due to acute vessel closure after this procedure. PTCA is judged a success if the arterial lumen at the stenosis is increased to more than 50% of the normal coronary artery diameter.

Restenosis at the site of the PTCA occurs within 6 months of the procedure in 30% of patients. Restenosis can be caused by elastic recoil of the vessel or by **intimal hyperplasia**, a thickening of the inner layer of the artery which is initiated by endothelial denudation, and which involves proliferation of intimal smooth muscle cells and the production of connective tissue. Restenosis generally causes a return of cardiac ischaemia and angina, in which case PTCA is repeated or CABG is performed.

Stents were first introduced in 1986 in an attempt to prevent elastic recoil and restenosis. Stents are cylindrical metal (e.g. stainless steel, platinum) mesh or slotted tubes that are implanted into the artery at the site of balloon expansion following angioplasty. They are mainly used in vessels > 3 mm in diameter and are designed either to be self-expanding, or to be expanded by the catheter balloon, so that they press out against the inner wall of the coronary artery, holding it open. Stenting is currently being used in ~90% of PTCA procedures as its introduction has substantially improved acute PTCA success, has reduced the rate of restenosis to ~15%, and has correspondingly decreased the need for repeat revascularizations. Various approaches are being tried to reduce this 'in-stent' restenosis still further. Notably, the 2002 RAVEL trial assessed the use of stents that were coated with the proliferation-inhibiting drug **rapamycin** (sirolimus), which gradually eluted from the stent over a month. Rapamycin caused a dramatic decrease in restenosis, and virtually abolished the need for another revascularization over the year following the procedure.

The main potential complication arising from stenting is thrombosis, and this can be well controlled with aspirin and clopidogrel.

Revascularization vs medical management: which patients benefit?

In general, revascularization is preferred for patients who are at high risk of developing worsening ischaemic heart disease and/or acute coronary syndromes, and also in those who have ischaemic symptoms (e.g. angina) which are not responding well to pharmacological ('medical') treatment, or in whom drugs cause intolerable side effects. Particularly important indications for revascularization in *stable angina* include the presence of significant plaques in three coronary arteries (particularly when the left anterior descending, which perfuses the largest fraction of the myocardium, is involved) and reduced left ventricular function, which indicates the presence of chronic ongoing ischaemia.

Revascularization is also very frequently used in *UA/NSTEMI* (see Chapter 38), and is recommended for patients who are judged to be at moderate or high risk for death or myocardial infarction, as judged by various indices relating to the seriousness of their signs and symptoms. Revascularization is also used in *acute myocardial infarction* (STEMI, see Chapters 41, 42) if thrombolysis is seen not to cause the desired reperfusion, or in patients who are developing cardiogenic shock. In *heart failure*, revascularization can be used to reperfuse a region of 'hibernating myocardium', in which cells are still alive but are contracting poorly because they are chronically ischaemic.

PTCA vs CABG

PTCA is preferred when one or two arteries are diseased, as long as the disease is not too diffuse and the plaques are amenable to this approach. CABG is used when all three main coronary arteries are diseased (triple vessel disease), when the left coronary mainstem has a significant stenosis, when the lesion is not amenable to PTCA, and when left ventricular function is poor. CABG has been shown to reduce angina symptoms more than does PTCA in the first 5 years after the procedure, but symptoms tend to return gradually over the years in either case, and eventually recur similarly after both procedures. Revascularization must be repeated much more often after PTCA compared to CABG, although improvements in stenting will probably narrow this difference.

Benefits of revascularization

Compared with medical therapy, CABG improves survival in patients with severe atherosclerotic disease in all three major coronary arteries or a more than 50% stenosis of the left main coronary artery, particularly if left ventricular function is impaired. Compared to medical therapy, PTCA does not improve survival. However, PTCA results in a greater improvement of angina symptoms and exercise tolerance than does medical therapy, and also diminishes the need for drugs.

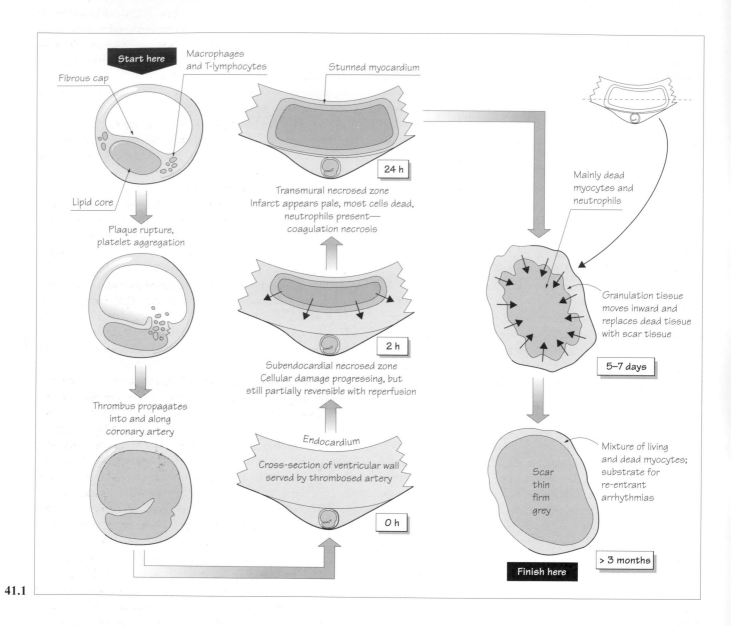

41.1

Infarction is tissue death caused by ischaemia. Acute **myocardial infarction** (MI) occurs when localized myocardial ischaemia causes the development of a defined region of **necrosis**. MI is most often caused by rupture of an atherosclerotic lesion in a coronary artery. This causes the formation of a thrombus that plugs the artery, stopping it from supplying blood to the region of the heart that it supplies.

Role of thrombosis in MI
Pivotal studies by DeWood and colleagues showed that *coronary thrombosis* is the critical event resulting in MI. Of patients presenting within 4 h of symptom onset with ECG evidence of transmural MI, coronary angiography showed that 87% had complete thrombotic occlusion of the infarct-related artery. The incidence of total occlusion fell to 65% 12–24 h after symptom onset due to spontaneous fibrinolysis. Fresh thrombi on top of ruptured plaques have also been demonstrated in the infarct-related arteries in patients dying of MI.

Mechanisms and consequences of plaque rupture
Coronary plaques which are prone to rupture are typically small and nonobstructive, with a large lipid-rich core covered by a thin fibrous cap. Activated **macrophages** and **T-lymphocytes** localized at the site of plaque rupture are thought to release **metalloproteases** and **cytokines** which weaken the fibrous cap, rendering it liable to tear or erode due to the shear stress exerted by the bloodflow.

Plaque rupture reveals subendothelial collagen, which serves as a site of platelet adhesion, activation and aggregation. This results in:

1 The release of substances such as *thromboxane A$_2$ (TXA$_2$)*, *fibrinogen, 5-hydroxytryptamine (5-HT), platelet activating factor* and *ADP*, which further promote platelet aggregation.
2 Activation of the clotting cascade, leading to fibrin formation and propagation and stabilization of the occlusive thrombus.

The endothelium is often damaged around areas of coronary artery disease. The resulting deficit of antithrombotic factors such as *thrombomodulin* and *prostacyclin* enhances thrombus formation. In addition, the tendency of several platelet-derived factors (e.g. TXA$_2$, 5-HT) to cause vasoconstriction is increased in the absence of endothelial-derived relaxing factors. This may promote the development of local vasospasm, which worsens coronary occlusion.

Sudden death and acute coronary syndrome onset show a **circadian variation** (daily cycle), peaking at around 9 a.m. with a trough at around 11 p.m. Levels of catecholamines peak about an hour after awakening in the morning, resulting in maximal levels of platelet aggregability, vascular tone, heart rate and blood pressure, which may trigger plaque rupture and thrombosis. Increased physical and mental stress can also cause MI and sudden death, supporting a role for increases in catecholamines in MI pathophysiology. Furthermore, chronic β-adrenergic receptor blockade abolishes the circadian rhythm of MI.

Autopsies of young subjects killed in road accidents often show small plaque ruptures in susceptible arteries, suggesting that plaque rupture does not always have pathological consequences. The degree of coronary occlusion and myocardial damage caused by plaque rupture probably depends on systemic catecholamine levels, as well as local factors such as plaque location and morphology, the depth of plaque rupture, and the extent to which coronary vasoconstriction occurs.

Severe and prolonged ischaemia produces a region of necrosis spanning the entire thickness of the myocardial wall. Such a *transmural* infarct usually causes ST segment elevation (i.e. STEMI, see Chapter 38). Less severe and protracted ischaemia can arise when:

1 Coronary occlusion is followed by spontaneous reperfusion.
2 The infarct-related artery is not completely occluded.
3 Occlusion is complete, but an existing collateral blood supply prevents complete ischaemia.
4 The oxygen demand in the affected zone of myocardium is smaller.

Under these conditions, the necrotic zone may be mainly limited to the subendocardium, typically causing non-ST segment elevation MI.

The classification of acute MI according to the presence or absence of ST segment elevation is designed to allow rapid decision-making concerning whether thrombolysis should be initiated (see Chapter 42). This classification replaces the previous one, based on the presence or absence of Q waves on the ECG, which was less useful for guiding immediate therapy. At c

Evolution of the infarct

Both infarcted and unaffected myocardial regions undergo progressive changes over the hours, days and weeks following coronary thrombosis. This process of postinfarct myocardial evolution leads to the occurrence of characteristic complications at predictable times after the initial event (see Chapter 42).

Ischaemia causes an immediate loss of contractility in the affected myocardium, a condition termed **hypokinesis**. Necrosis starts to develop in the subendocardium (which is most prone to ischaemia; see Chapter 37), about 15–30 min after coronary occlusion. The necrotic region grows outward towards the epicardium over the next 3–6 h, eventually spanning the entire ventricular wall. In some areas (generally at the edges of the infarct) the myocardium is **stunned** (reversibly damaged) and will eventually recover if bloodflow is restored. Contractility in the remaining viable myocardium increases, a process termed **hyperkinesis**.

A progression of cellular, histological and gross changes develop within the infarct. Although alterations in the gross appearance of infarcted tissue are not apparent for at least 6 h after the onset of cell death, cell biochemistry and ultrastructure begin to show abnormalities within 20 min. Cell damage is progressive, becomingly increasingly irreversible over about 12 h. This period therefore provides a window of opportunity during which thrombolysis and reperfusion may salvage some of the infarct (see Chapter 43).

Between 4 and 12 h after cell death starts, the infarcted myocardium begins to undergo **coagulation necrosis**, a process characterized by cell swelling, organelle breakdown and protein denaturation. After about 18 h, **neutrophils** (phagocytic lymphocytes) enter the infarct. Their numbers reach a peak after about 5 days, and then decline. After 3–4 days, **granulation tissue** appears at the edges of the infarct zone. This consists of **macrophages**, **fibroblasts**, which lay down scar tissue, and **new capillaries**. The infarcted myocardium is especially soft between 4 and 7 days, and is therefore maximally prone to **rupturing**. This event is usually fatal, may occur at any time during the first 2 weeks and is responsible for about 10% of MI mortality. As the granulation tissue migrates inward toward the centre of the infarct over several weeks, the necrotic tissue is engulfed and digested by the macrophages. The granulation tissue then progressively matures, with an increase in connective (scar) tissue and loss of capillaries. After 2–3 months, the infarct has healed, leaving a noncontracting region of the ventricular wall that is thinned, firm and pale grey.

Infarct expansion, the stretching and thinning of the infarcted wall, may occur within the first day or so after a MI, especially if the infarction is large or transmural, or has an anterior location. Over the course of several months, there is progressive dilatation, not only of the infarct zone, but also of healthy myocardium. This process of **ventricular remodelling** is caused by an increase in end-diastolic wall stress. Infarct expansion puts patients at a sub-stantial risk for the development of congestive heart failure, ventricular arrhythmias, and free wall rupture.

42 Clinical aspects of acute myocardial infarction

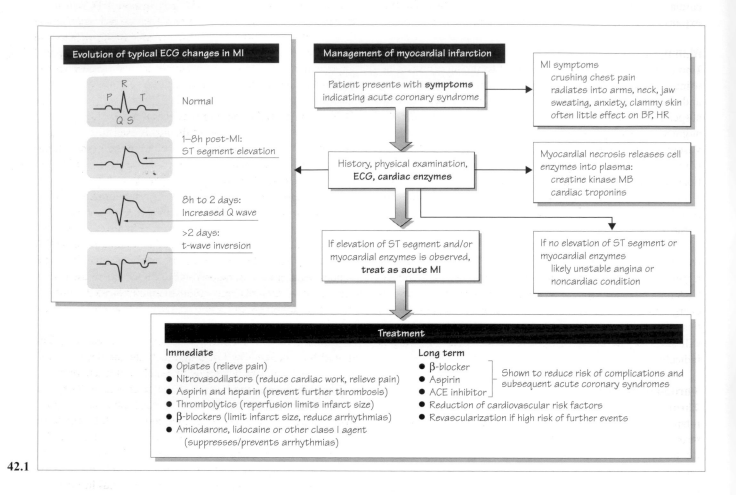

Evolution of typical ECG changes in MI

R
P   T
Q S
Normal

1–8h post-MI:
ST segment elevation

8h to 2 days:
Increased Q wave

>2 days:
t-wave inversion

Management of myocardial infarction

Patient presents with **symptoms** indicating acute coronary syndrome

MI symptoms
crushing chest pain
radiates into arms, neck, jaw
sweating, anxiety, clammy skin
often little effect on BP, HR

History, physical examination, **ECG, cardiac enzymes**

Myocardial necrosis releases cell enzymes into plasma:
creatine kinase MB
cardiac troponins

If elevation of ST segment and/or myocardial enzymes is observed, **treat as acute MI**

If no elevation of ST segment or myocardial enzymes
likely unstable angina or noncardiac condition

Treatment

Immediate
- Opiates (relieve pain)
- Nitrovasodilators (reduce cardiac work, relieve pain)
- Aspirin and heparin (prevent further thrombosis)
- Thrombolytics (reperfusion limits infarct size)
- β-blockers (limit infarct size, reduce arrhythmias)
- Amiodarone, lidocaine or other class I agent (suppresses/prevents arrhythmias)

Long term
- β-blocker ⎤
- Aspirin   ⎥ Shown to reduce risk of complications and
- ACE inhibitor ⎦ subsequent acute coronary syndromes
- Reduction of cardiovascular risk factors
- Revascularization if high risk of further events

42.1

Symptoms and signs

Patients present with central crushing chest pain, which may radiate into the arms, jaw or neck. The pain lasts > 30 min and is not relieved by nitroglycerin. The patient is frequently sweating and may appear cold and clammy. Nausea or vomiting and intense feelings of anxiety are common. Some individuals present atypically, with no symptoms (**silent infarction**, most common in diabetic subjects), unusual locations of the pain, syncope or peripheral embolization. The pulse may demonstrate a tachycardia or bradycardia. The blood pressure is usually normal. However, a systolic pressure of < 90 mmHg and evidence of organ hypoperfusion herald **cardiogenic shock**, where cardiac output is insufficient for adequate tissue perfusion. The rest of the examination of the cardiovascular system may be remarkably normal, but there may be a third or fourth sound audible on auscultation as well as a systolic murmur.

Investigations

ECG changes associated with MI indicate the site, extent and thickness of the infarct. ST segment abnormalities, increased Q waves and inversion of the T wave typically evolve in transmural MI (i.e. STEMI) as shown in Fig. 42.1. A more than twofold elevation of plasma concentrations of cardiac cellular enzymes indicates that myocardial necrosis has occurred. These include **creatine kinase MB** (CK-MB) and **cardiac troponins T and I**. CK-MB levels begin to rise within 4–8 h, peak at 24 h, and decline to normal at 2–3 days. The cardiac troponins begin to rise within 4–8 h and remain elevated for 4–7 days.

Complications

With large infarctions (> 20–25% of the left ventricle (LV)), depression of pump function is sufficient to cause **cardiac failure**. An infarction involving > 40% of the LV causes cardiogenic shock. **Rupture** of the free LV wall (see Chapter 41) is almost always fatal. Rupture of the ventricular septum may result in leakage of blood between the ventricles. Rupture of the myocardium underlying a papillary muscle, or more rarely of the papillary muscle itself, may cause **mitral regurgitation. Arrhythmias** in the acute phase include ventricular ectopic beats, ventricular tachycardia or ventricular fibrillation. Supraventricular arrhythmias include atrial ectopics, flutter and fibrillation. Bradyarrhythmias are also common, including sinus bradycardia, and first-, second- and third-degree AV block. **Infarct expansion** (see Chapter 41) is a dangerous late complication.

Management

Immediate: Patients with suspected MI should be assessed using a 12-lead ECG, and by brief history and examination, and should be put on bed rest and oxygen. All patients with suspected MI should receive **aspirin** to block further platelet aggregation. **Opiates** are generally used to relieve pain. **Nitrovasodilators** may also help to reduce cardiac work and control pain. **β-blockers** should be used unless there are contraindications (e.g. LV failure). Patients with ST elevation of more than 1 mm in two contiguous leads (indicates STEMI), or new left bundle branch block, should undergo **thrombolysis**.

Subsequent: Long-term treatment with aspirin, β-blockers and **ACE inhibitors** reduces both the complications of MI and the risk of reinfarction. Cessation of smoking, treatment of hypertension and diabetes, and reduction of lipids using HMG-CoA reductase inhibitors (see Chapter 33) are vital. Prior to discharge from hospital, patients are given an exercise stress test. If this indicates that the risk of further events is high, or if they are still suffering from angina attacks, early revascularization is indicated.

Thrombolytic agents

Thrombolysis is the dissolution of the blood clot plugging the infarct-related coronary artery. As described in Chapter 43, thrombolytic agents induce **fibrinolysis**, the fragmentation of the fibrin strands which hold the clot together. This leads to *reperfusion* of the infarct zone. Reperfusion limits infarct size and reduces the risk of complications such as infarct expansion, arrhythmias and cardiac failure. Clinical trials, notably ISIS-2 (1988), have demonstrated that thrombolytic agents reduce mortality by about 25% in STEMI, although patients without ST elevation (indicates NSTEMI) do *not* benefit from thrombolysis. It is critical that thrombolysis is instituted as quickly as possible. Although significant reductions in short-term mortality occur when thrombolytics are given within 12 h of symptom onset, the greatest benefits occur when therapy is instituted within 3 h.

The two agents mainly used for thrombolysis are **streptokinase (SK)** and **tissue plasminogen activator (tPA)** (see Chapter 43). tPA appears to have a slight survival benefit compared to SK, but the latter is much less expensive and therefore more widely used. Both agents are given by infusion. tPA is very quickly cleared from the plasma, and **reteplase** and **tenecteplase** are newer agents that have been made by modifying the structure of tPA in such as way as to retard plasma clearance. Both can therefore be given by bolus injection, thus facilitating prehospital thrombolysis.

The main risk of thrombolysis is bleeding, particularly intracerebral haemorrhage (stroke), although the latter occurs in only ~0.5% of cases. Contraindications to thrombolytic therapy include prior stroke, active ulcers and recent surgery.

If thrombolysis fails to provide reperfusion, **PTCA** is used. Immediate PTCA is also an alternative to pharmacological thrombolysis, and indeed has been shown to be superior to it in providing reperfusion and increasing survival. Its widespread implementation is, however, presently limited by cost and by the need for it to be carried out by experienced staff.

Other drugs used in acute myocardial infarction

Antiplatelet and **anticoagulant** therapy is used after MI to prevent further platelet aggregation and thrombosis in the infarct-related artery. **Aspirin** inhibits platelet aggregation (see Chapter 43). ISIS-2 demonstrated a 23% reduction in 35-day mortality in patients randomized to 160 mg/day of aspirin. Combined aspirin and SK had an additive benefit compared to placebo (42% reduction); 160–325 mg of aspirin should be given daily to all patients to prevent vessel occlusion and infarction. Because tPA is more fibrin specific and has a shorter half-life than SK, intravenous heparin for a duration of 48–72 h should be used when this agent is administered. Unless contraindicated, subcutaneous low-dose heparin should be used in MI patients to prevent deep vein thrombosis and pulmonary emboli.

β-blockers are beneficial in MI for several reasons. They diminish O_2 demand by lowering heart rate and decrease ventricular wall stress by lowering afterload. β-blockers therefore reduce ischaemia and infarct size when given acutely. They also decrease recurrent ischaemia and free wall rupture and suppress arrhythmias (see Chapter 48). Long-term oral β-blockade reduces mortality, recurrent MI and sudden death by about 25%.

ACE inhibitors reduce afterload and ventricular wall stress and improve ejection fraction. Inhibition of ACE raises bradykinin levels, which may improve endothelial function and limit coronary vasospasm. ACE inhibitors also limit ventricular remodelling and infarct expansion (see Chapter 41), thereby reducing mortality and the incidence of congestive heart failure and recurrent MI. Therapy should be instituted immediately in patients with STEMI or evidence of heart failure, and should continue long term if evidence of LV dysfunction is present.

Severe LV failure as a result of MI is heralded by a large fall in cardiac output, pulmonary congestion and often hypotension. Treatment involves O_2 to prevent hypoxaemia, a diuretic to reduce preload, and nitroglycerin (glyceryl trinitrate) to reduce afterload. Revascularization is crucial. If ventricular failure is severe (cardiogenic shock), **intraortic balloon counterpulsation** can be used temporarily to support the circulation. A catheter-mounted balloon is inserted via the common femoral artery and positioned in the descending thoracic aorta. The balloon is inflated during diastole, increasing the pressure in the aortic arch and thereby improving perfusion of the coronary and cerebral arteries. During systole, deflation of the balloon creates a suction effect which reduces ventricular afterload and promotes systemic perfusion.

43 Anticoagulants and thrombolytics

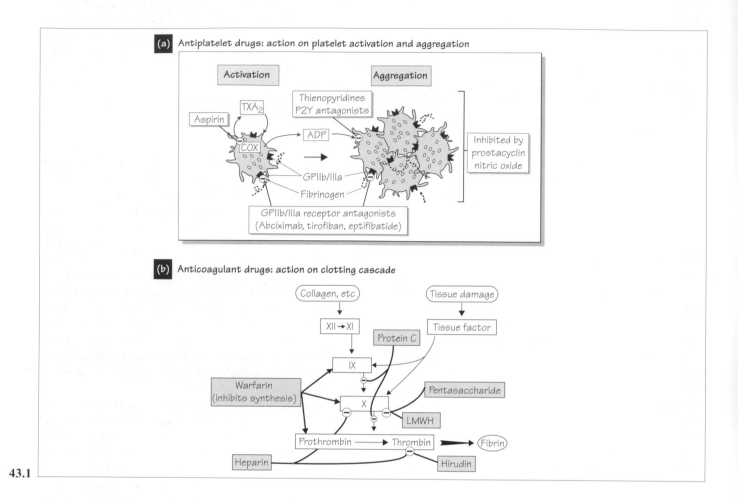

(a) Antiplatelet drugs: action on platelet activation and aggregation

(b) Anticoagulant drugs: action on clotting cascade

43.1

Thrombosis and embolism are the main cause of death in the Western world, often as a result of **atherosclerotic plaque rupture** in acute coronary syndromes, or **thromboembolism**, particular pulmonary embolism, following deep vein thrombosis (DVT). Arterial (white, platelet-rich) thrombi are primarily treated with antiplatelet drugs and thrombolytics, whilst venous (red) thrombi are primarily treated with anticoagulants. All anticoagulant and thrombolytic therapies increase the risk of bleeding, and depending on type may be contraindicated in patients with prior stroke, active ulcers, pregnancy or recent surgery.

Antiplatelet drugs

Aspirin (*acetylsalicylic acid*) is the most important antiplatelet drug. It irreversibly inhibits **cyclooxygenase** (COX), the first enzyme in the sequence leading to the formation of **thromboxane A_2** (TXA$_2$) and **prostacyclin** (PGI$_2$). TXA$_2$ synthesized in platelets is a key platelet activator (see Chapter 7), whereas endothelium-derived prostacyclin inhibits platelet activation and aggregation by increasing cAMP. Although aspirin blocks

the formation of both TXA$_2$ and prostacyclin, its effect on platelet TXA$_2$ production predominates. This selectivity arises because aspirin inhibits COX *irreversibly*, and so prostacyclin and TXA$_2$ levels can only recover when new COX is produced via gene transcription. This cannot occur in the platelets, which lack nuclei (see Chapter 5). TXA$_2$ production therefore remains depressed for several days, until new platelets are formed. Conversely, endothelial cells can make new COX within hours. Aspirin therapy therefore produces a sustained increase in the prostacyclin : TXA$_2$ ratio, thereby inhibiting platelet activation and aggregation. **Side effects/risks:** Gastrointestinal problems and haemorrhage. **Emerging therapy:** A potentially promising development is nitroaspirin, a combination of aspirin with an NO-releasing moiety. NO also inhibits platelet aggregation, and nitroaspirin is reported to be better tolerated in terms of GI tract problems.

The *thienopyridine* derivatives **clopidogrel** and **ticlopidine** inhibit *ADP-induced* platelet aggregation via an active metabolite, and take > 24 h to reach maximal effect. They are particularly useful for aspirin-intolerant patients and in preventing thrombi formation on new coronary artery stents (see Chapter 38). Long-term treatment with clopidogrel plus aspirin is reported to be beneficial in acute coronary syndromes. **Side effects/risks:** Rash; ticlopidine (but not clopidogrel) may cause neutropenia. **Emerging therapy:** Direct antagonists of ADP (P2Y) receptors are in phase III clinical trials. These have a potential advantage over thienopyridines of rapidity of action, and possibly complete inhibition of ADP-mediated effects.

Glycoprotein IIb/IIIa receptors expressed on platelets following activation bind fibrinogen and vWF, promoting aggregation (see Chapter 7). The monoclonal antibody **abciximab** and peptides **tirofiban** and **eptifibatide** interfere with binding to GPIIb/IIIa receptors, and thus inhibit aggregation. In patients with unstable angina or undergoing high-risk angioplasty, the addition of GPIIb/IIIa blockade to aspirin and heparin significantly reduces short-term mortality, MI and need for urgent bypass surgery or revascularization.

Anticoagulant drugs

Heparin (*unfractionated* heparin) is a mixture of mucopolysaccharides derived from mast cells. It activates **antithrombin III** (a serine protease inhibitor), which inhibits thrombin and factor X, as well as factors IX, XI and XII (see Chapter 7). Inhibition of thrombin requires heparin binding to thrombin and antithrombin III; inhibition of factor X requires binding to antithrombin III alone. Unfractionated heparin is inactivated by **platelet factor 4**, and has large variability of action with dose due to variable protein binding; an *in vitro* clotting test is required to set dosing correctly. Intravenous heparin is immediately effective but has a relatively short half-life (< 90 min). Approximately 10% of patients on heparin develop thrombocytopenia.

Low molecular weight heparins (LMWHs; e.g. *enoxaparin*) are ~30% the molecular weight of unfractionated heparin. LMWHs bind only to antithrombin III and not thrombin, and are therefore more effective at inhibiting factor X. LMWHs are given subcutaneously. There is minimal protein binding, little inactivation by platelet factor 4, and a longer half-life, resulting in predictable dose responses and no need for routine clotting tests. The likelihood of thrombocytopenia is much reduced. LMWHs have largely replaced unfractionated heparin in clinical use.

Warfarin (coumarin, dicoumarol) is the most important oral anticoagulant, and acts as a vitamin K antagonist, thereby inhibiting production of prothrombin and factors VII, IX and X by the liver. As such it is only effective *in vivo*. Although slow in onset (~1–2 days), warfarin can provide effective support for ~5 days. Numerous factors including disease and drugs affect the sensitivity to warfarin, and it is therefore monitored routinely by measurement of **prothrombin time** (see Chapter 7), expressed as the *International Normalized Ratio* (**INR**); the dose is normally adjusted to give an INR of ~3.

Emerging therapies: Several novel anticoagulant therapies are in phase III trials. **Pentasaccharide**, a small synthetic, heparin-like inhibitor of factor X, has been shown to be more effective than LMWH in suppressing the rate of DVT after orthopaedic surgery, and shows great promise. Likewise, initial results suggest that recombinant thrombomodulin and protein C are effective. Trials of **hirudin**, a direct inhibitor of thrombin, have, however, been disappointing.

Thrombolytics

Thrombolysis is dissolution of the blood clot. In coronary artery disease this allows reperfusion of the infarct zone, so limiting infarct size and reducing complications. The greatest benefits of thrombolytic therapy occur when it is instituted within 3 h, although there are reductions in short-term mortality when it is given within 12 h. Thrombolytics only have proven efficacy in arterial thrombosis, and because of the risk of gut and intracerebral haemorrhage (stroke) are only used for venous thrombosis in life-threatening pulmonary embolism. Thrombolytic (**fibrinolytic**) agents act by inducing **fibrinolysis**, the breakdown of fibrin strands holding the clot together. Fibrinolysis occurs when **plasminogen** is converted to the fibrinolytic enzyme **plasmin** by **tissue plasminogen activator (tPA)**. Plasmin also inactivates fibrinogen and coagulation factors V and VIII (see Chapter 7).

Streptokinase (SK) is a *Streptococcus* bacterial protein that is inactive until it binds to plasminogen. This complex then cleaves other plasminogen molecules to produce plasmin. SK has a plasma clearance time of 15–25 min. It activates plasminogen not only within clots but also in the plasma, and so can cause haemorrhage. SK can only be used once since it induces antibodies that block its action and may cause an allergic reaction on second application. **Anistreplase** (APSAC) is a complex of human plasminogen and SK that is rendered inactive by the addition of an anisoyl group to the streptokinase. This group is removed slowly in plasma, freeing SK to activate plasminogen. Similar to SK, APSAC is antigenic and may cause allergic reactions. APSAC has a long plasma clearance time of 50–90 min. Aspirin in combination with SK has a *synergistic benefit* on reducing mortality.

Recombinant **tPA** (*alteplase*) binds to fibrin, so it has a greater effect on clot-associated plasminogen than on plasma plasminogen; it is not antigenic. tPA is cleared from plasma within 4–8 min, and must therefore be given by intravenous infusion; **reteplase**, another recombinant version of tPA, has a longer clearance time and can be given as a bolus. **uPA** (*urokinase*) is another endogenous plasminogen activator.

44 Chronic heart failure

(a) Left ventricular function curve

Effect of reduced contractility in heart failure

Stroke volume

Normal exercise

Normal rest

Normal — Mild failure — Severe

End diastolic pressure (stretch)

Exercise — Normal

Rest

Exercise — Failure
Rest

Severe failure

1 2 3

(c) Role of compensatory mechanisms in progression of heart failure

↓Cardiac output

Sympathetic activation

Renin–angiotensin activation

α β

Direct effect of norepinephrine

↑Energy deficit
↑Ca²⁺ overload
↑Myocardial damage
↑Cardiac remodelling

Direct effect of angiotensin II

↑Contractility and heart rate

↑Work

Aldosterone

↑Afterload

↑Preload

Renal artery

Fluid retention

Arterial vasoconstriction

Angiotensin II

(b) Origin of major symptoms and signs in heart failure

Exercise intolerance

Fatigue, weakness

Peripheral vasoconstriction

LV failure — CO

↑HR contractility

Neurohumoral compensation

Na⁺ water retention

↑LVEDP

Starling's Law

↑CVP

Dyspnoea
Pulmonary oedema
Dilated heart

↑Load on RV
RV failure

Peripheral oedema
Hepatomegaly
Ascites

Underlying causes of heart failure

Primary defect	Examples
Myocardial dysfunction	Ischaemic heart disease. Pregnancy, congenital cardiomyopathies. Myocardial disease e.g. amyloidosis
Volume overload	Aortic or mitral valve regurgitation
Pressure overload	Aortic stenosis, hypertension
Impaired filling	Constrictive pericarditis: rheumatic heart disease. Cardiac tamponade: excess fluid pressure in pericardial space
Arrhythmias	Atrial fibrillation
High output	Thyrotoxicosis, arteriovenous shunts, anaemia

44.1

In **heart failure**, the heart is unable to produce an adequate cardiac output to perfuse the tissues, or can do so only with an elevated filling pressure (**preload**). Initially, adaptive mechanisms may compensate and so maintain cardiac output at rest, although they may not be sufficient during exercise. In spite of these mechanisms cardiac function eventually declines, and heart failure becomes severe (**decompensated**). This can be precipitated by other acute diseases or stress. Heart failure occurs in ~2–3% of the general population but increases with age; prevalence is > 10% in patients over 65 years. Survival is ~50% over 5 years.

Systolic failure is a defect in function that impairs ejection, whereas **diastolic failure** is a defect in ventricular filling. These often coexist, particularly in ischaemic heart disease.

Clinical manifestations of heart failure

Patients generally present with **dyspnoea** (breathlessness), though initially only during exercise, also weakness, fatigue and **peripheral oedema** (fluid retention in tissues; see Chapter 20), most commonly seen as swollen legs. The heart and liver are enlarged, and a high CVP distends the jugular veins. A **gallop**

rhythm may be heard due to high cardiac filling pressure (see Chapter 13). Cardiac output and BP may be normal in moderate heart failure, but the **ejection fraction** (proportion of end-diastolic volume ejected per beat) is always reduced.

Pathophysiology of chronic heart failure

Major causes of heart failure are shown in the table in Fig. 44.1. The most common is **ischaemic heart disease**, when coronary flow and oxygen delivery to cardiac muscle are insufficient. **Contractility** (see Chapter 14) is reduced, and the ventricular function curve is depressed (Fig. 44.1a). In mild failure, output can only be obtained at rest with increased end-diastolic pressure (EDP) (**1**). In exercise the function curve may never reach the required output (**2**); the increase in contractility is small because sympathetic tone is already high (see below). In severe, decompensated failure, normal resting output cannot be obtained even with substantial increases in EDP (**3**).

Left heart failure: Ischaemic heart disease most commonly affects the left ventricle. Decreased output leads to an increased left ventricular EDP (preload) and pulmonary venous pressure as blood 'backs up' in the pulmonary circulation (**pulmonary congestion**; Fig. 44.1b). This causes the heart to **dilate**, and the increased pulmonary capillary pressure promotes fluid accumulation in the lung interstitium (see Chapter 20). The increased blood and fluid in the lungs makes them stiff, causing **dyspnoea**. Dyspnoea may only occur when the patient lies down (**orthopnoea**) as fluid redistributes to the lungs. Episodic dyspnoea causing waking at night is called **paroxysmal dyspnoea**. A severe rise in capillary pressure causes fluid to enter the alveoli (**pulmonary oedema**), a life-threatening condition causing extreme dyspnoea, reduced gas exchange and hypoxaemia.

Right heart failure: Left heart failure increases pulmonary vascular pressure, and can therefore lead to pressure overload and failure of the right heart, a situation called **congestive heart failure** (Fig. 44.1b). Right heart failure alone can be caused by chronic lung disease (**cor pulmonale**), pulmonary hypertension or embolism, and valve disease. CVP is greatly increased in right heart failure, seen as **distension of the jugular veins**, and leads to fluid accumulation in the peripheral tissues (**peripheral oedema**), peritoneum (**ascites**) and **liver**, causing tenderness and enlargement (**hepatomegaly**). Ambulatory patients show **pitting oedema** of the ankles (a depression is left following compression with a finger), which is relieved on lying down.

Compensatory mechanisms

Adaptive mechanisms initially compensate for reduced function, but are often deleterious when sustained. They all increase cardiac work and thus oxygen requirement, which is clearly detrimental in ischaemic heart disease.

Starling's Law: Reduced output and ejection fraction increase preload (see above). Cardiac force therefore increases due to **Starling's Law**, partially restoring output (Fig. 44.1a,b; see

Chapter 14), but at the expense of a maintained increase in filling pressure.

Neurohumoral system: Low blood pressure initiates the **baroreceptor reflex**, and stimulates the sympathetic nervous system (Fig. 44.1b; see Chapter 27). This increases heart rate (**tachycardia**) and contractility, and improves cardiac output (see Chapters 11, 14). Venoconstriction increases CVP, and systemic vasoconstriction increases total peripheral resistance (TPR) which helps maintain BP. Afterload is, however, increased, and the redistribution of output from the skeletal muscle and splanchnic circulations leads to muscle weakness and fatigue, and impaired renal function. These effects may be limited in late disease because β-adrenoceptor density falls, and norepinephrine sensitivity decreases. Vasoconstriction of renal arteries (Fig. 44.1b) reduces filtration and urine production (**oliguria**), and causes the release of **renin**. Renin activates **angiotensin I**, which is converted to **angiotensin II**, a powerful vasoconstrictor that also potentiates sympathetic activity. Angiotensin II stimulates the adrenal glands to produce **aldosterone**, which augments Na^+ and hence water reabsorption, thus increasing blood volume and CVP. **Vasopressin** (ADH) also increases, leading to further water retention.

Myocardial hypertrophy: A sustained increase in load leads to a rise in ventricular wall thickness as the muscle cells grow larger (**myocardial hypertrophy**); this is common in pressure overload-induced failure, but not in ischaemic heart disease. Although hypertrophy improves the contractile force, the thicker ventricle is less **compliant** (flexible) and stretches less as EDP rises; Starling's Law is therefore less effective. Capillaries are also further apart (**capillary density** falls), increasing diffusion distance and reducing **coronary reserve** (difference between maximum and resting coronary flow). Perfusion is therefore reduced in exercise. Changes in contractile protein isoforms (myosin, tropomyosin) also decrease contraction velocity and contractility. Gross hypertrophy may physically impair valve operation.

Exacerbation of cardiac dysfunction

An important component of the transition to full heart failure is a gradual reduction in myocardial function as a direct result of the compensatory mechanisms (Fig. 44.1c). All factors increasing work will contribute to any **energy deficit**, and continued stimulation by norepinephrine and angiotensin II promotes cellular Ca^{2+} **overload**. This causes further cell damage and necrosis, and fosters the generation of arrhythmias.

Cardiac dilatation during failure reduces its *efficiency* to develop ventricular pressure because of the **Law of Laplace**, which states that pressure in a sphere is proportional to wall tension divided by radius. Large, dilated hearts therefore have to contract harder in order to develop the same pressure as smaller hearts. This becomes a major problem in the grossly dilated, failing heart.

45 Treatment of chronic heart failure

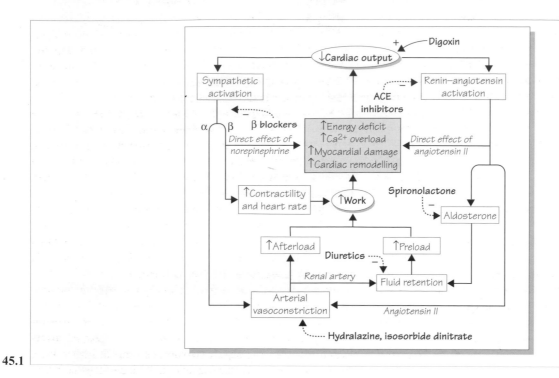

45.1

Therapy of chronic heart failure (CHF) is designed to: (i) improve the quality of life by reducing symptoms; (ii) lengthen survival; and (iii) slow the progression of cardiac deterioration. CHF typically has an underlying cause such as ischaemic heart disease, and may be exacerbated by specific **precipitating factors** such as infection or arrhythmias, as well as by myocardial abnormalities which develop as CHF progresses (e.g. valvular dysfunction). In addition to treating the symptoms of CHF *per se*, both underlying and precipitating factors should, if possible, be treated. Restricting activity and reducing dietary sodium help to lessen cardiac workload and fluid retention.

The **sympathetic** and **renin–angiotensin–aldosterone** systems activated in response to reduced pump function initially help to maintain cardiac output, but also drive the progression of cardiac deterioration (Fig. 45.1; see also Chapter 44). Therapy increasingly involves inhibiting these systems. It is currently recommended that treatment of CHF is initiated with **angiotensin-converting enzyme inhibitors (ACE-I)**, which slow CHF progression, lengthen survival time and improve haemodynamic parameters. **Angiotensin receptor blockers (ARBs)** are used as an alternative in patients who cannot tolerate ACE-I. A **diuretic** can also be used to control fluid accumulation. Once the patient has stabilized on this treatment, a **β-blocker** can be added in gradually increasing doses. **Digoxin** is often used to support cardiac function and reduce symptoms.

In severe or refractory CHF, or when existing therapy fails to control symptoms adequately, the aldosterone antagonist **spironolactone** can be used, as can vasodilators such as **hydralazine** and **isosorbide dinitrate**. Positive inotropes such as **dobutamine**, **dopamine** or **milrinone** may be used temporarily if decompensation occurs.

ACE-I and other vasodilators

As described in Chapter 28, angiotension II causes vasoconstriction and promotes fluid retention via multiple mechanisms. ACE-I, which inhibit the conversion of angiotensin I to angiotensin II, therefore dilate arteries and veins, and reduce blood volume and oedema. Arterial vasodilatation decreases afterload and cardiac work, and improves tissue perfusion by increasing stroke volume and cardiac output. Venous dilatation and reduction of fluid retention diminish pulmonary congestion, oedema and central venous pressure (CVP) (preload). Reduction of preload lowers ventricular filling pressure, therefore lowering cardiac wall stress, workload and ischaemia. ACE-I also delay abnormal cardiac hypertrophy and fibrosis, which are thought to be promoted by angiotensin II.

Angiotensin receptor blockers such as **losartan** are used in patients unable to tolerate the cough or renal dysfunction occasionally caused by ACE-I. The combination of the nitrovasodilator isosorbide dinitrate (see Chapter 39) and hydralazine can also prolong survival, although not as effect-ively as ACE-I. Hydralazine causes mainly arterial vasodila-tation, possibly via inhibition of Ca^{2+} release from the sarcoplasmic reticulum.

β-Receptor blockers

The 1993 MDC study reported that the β_1-selective antagonist **metoprolol** reduced mortality when added to conventional therapy for mild to moderate CHF. The benefits of adding metoprolol to standard therapy (ACE-I and diuretics) were confirmed in the 1999 MERIT-HF study, which showed that this drug reduced 1-year mortality by 34% in patients with mild to severe CHF. **Bisoprolol**, another β_1-selective antagonist, was shown by the 1999 CIBIS-II trial to similarly diminish mortality. **Carvedilol** is a nonselective β-blocker which has additional α-antagonist and antioxidant properties, and has also been shown to prolong survival in CHF. The 2003 COMET trial showed that when given to patients being treated with ACE-I and diuretics, carvedilol extended survival to a greater extent than did metoprolol.

Long-term treatment with β-blockers has been shown to increase ejection fraction, reduce systolic and diastolic volume, and eventually cause regression of left ventricular hypertrophy. Other beneficial effects of β-blockers in CHF probably include reduced ischaemia and a reduction in heart rate, thus improving myocardial perfusion, and inhibition of the deleterious effects of excess catecholamines on myocardial structure and metabolism. β-blockers appear to be particularly effective in reducing sudden death in those with CHF, suggesting that the prevention of *ventricular fibrillation* (see Chapter 48) constitutes an important part of their action.

The negative inotropic effect of β-blockers is potentially hazardous in some patients with CHF, since cardiac function is already compromised. Therapy is therefore initiated with low doses which are carefully elevated over several weeks or months.

Diuretics

Diuretics reduce fluid accumulation by increasing renal salt and water excretion. Preload, pulmonary congestion and systemic oedema are thereby relieved. **Loop diuretics** inhibit the Na^+–K^+–$2Cl^-$ symport in the thick ascending loop of Henle. Na^+ and Cl^- reabsorption is thereby inhibited, and the retention of these ions in the tubule promotes fluid loss in the urine. Diuretics are commonly used in CHF, and include **furosemide**, **bumetanide**, **piretanide**, **torasemide** and **ethacrynic acid**. Thiazide and thiazide-related diuretics (see Chapter 35) are also used to treat heart failure.

Both loop and thiazide diuretics can cause hypokalaemia and metabolic alkalosis because the increased Na^+ retained in the tubular fluid is partly exchanged for K^+ and H^+ in the distal nephron. This process is stimulated by aldosterone (see Chapter 28), and diuretic-induced hypokalaemia can be controlled by an ACE-I or **spironolactone**, an aldosterone antagonist. Hypokalaemia can also be treated with K^+ supplements, or the use of **K^+-sparing diuretics** such as **amiloride** or **triamterine**. These inhibit Na^+ reabsorption in the collecting duct. Long-term use of loop diuretics can result in hypovolaemia, reduced plasma Mg^{2+}, Ca^{2+} and Na^+, and hyperuricaemia and hyperglycaemia. This is more common in the elderly, who may require high doses of diuretics to overcome **diuretic resistance**.

Cardiac glycosides

Cardiac glycosides include ouabain, digitoxin and **digoxin**, which is used most widely. Digoxin improves CHF symptoms, but does not prolong life. Cardiac glycosides inhibit the Na^+ pump in cardiac muscle, thereby indirectly inhibiting the Na^+–Ca^{2+} antiport and thus increasing intracellular Ca^{2+} (see Chapter 11). The rise in Ca^{2+} enhances contractility and shortens action potential duration and refractory period in atrial and ventricular cells by stimulating K^+ channels. Digoxin has been shown to increase baroreceptor responsiveness, thereby reducing sympathetic tone.

Digoxin also acts on the nervous system to increase vagal tone. This slows both sinoatrial node activity and atrioventricular node (AVN) conduction, and can be useful in treating atrial arrhythmias (see Chapter 47). It is therefore mainly used in patients with both CHF and atrial fibrillation.

Even a small (2–3-fold) excess of digoxin over the optimal therapeutic concentration can cause arrhythmias. This occurs because an excessive rise in $[Ca^{2+}]_i$ causes oscillations in membrane potential after action potentials. These **delayed afterdepolarizations** can trigger ectopic beats, and at higher doses can trigger ventricular tachycardia. Inhibition of the Na^+ pump also decreases intracellular K^+, causing depolarization and facilitating arrhythmias. In addition, excess digoxin can increase vagal tone enough to block conduction at the AVN, and can also raise sympathetic tone, again favouring arrhythmias. Digoxin toxicity is enhanced by **hypokalaemia** (low plasma K^+), because K^+ decreases the affinity of digoxin for the Na^+ pump. Digoxin also causes toxic gastrointestinal effects, including anorexia, nausea and vomiting. Acute toxicity can be treated with intravenous K^+, antiarrhythmics (e.g. lidocaine) and digoxin-specific antibodies.

Spironolactone

Aldosterone levels initially fall during ACE-I treatment, but often rise again ('escape') during prolonged treatment. Aldosterone has a number of effects which worsen CHF and its consequences; these include inducing cardiac fibrosis, reducing nitric oxide release, and promoting arrhythmias by raising plasma K^+ and cardiac norepinephrine release.

The aldosterone antagonist **spironolactone** was shown in the 1999 RALES trial to reduce mortality when added to ACE-I in severe CHF. Very few of these patients were receiving β-blockers, and so it is not known whether spironolactone is of benefit in those already receiving ACE-I and β-blockers, or in less severe CHF. Spironolactone also causes antiandrogenic side effects such as gynaecomastia, and the more selective aldosterone antagonist **eplerenone** is currently under investigation as an alternative.

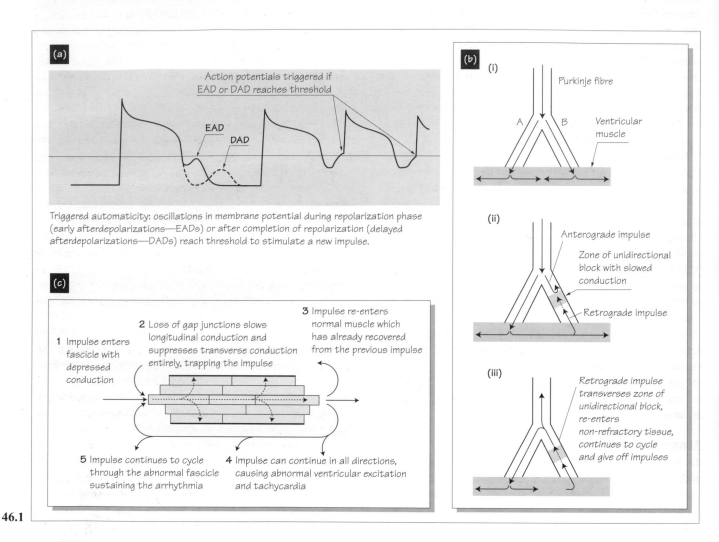

(a) Triggered automaticity: oscillations in membrane potential during repolarization phase (early afterdepolarizations—EADs) or after completion of repolarization (delayed afterdepolarizations—DADs) reach threshold to stimulate a new impulse.

Action potentials triggered if EAD or DAD reaches threshold

EAD
DAD

(b) (i) Purkinje fibre
A   B   Ventricular muscle

(ii) Anterograde impulse
Zone of unidirectional block with slowed conduction
Retrograde impulse

(iii) Retrograde impulse transverses zone of unidirectional block, re-enters non-refractory tissue, continues to cycle and give off impulses

(c)
1 Impulse enters fascicle with depressed conduction
2 Loss of gap junctions slows longitudinal conduction and suppresses transverse conduction entirely, trapping the impulse
3 Impulse re-enters normal muscle which has already recovered from the previous impulse
5 Impulse continues to cycle through the abnormal fascicle sustaining the arrhythmia
4 Impulse can continue in all directions, causing abnormal ventricular excitation and tachycardia

46.1

Arrhythmias are abnormalities of the heart rate or rhythm. These are caused by disorders of impulse generation or conduction.

Disorders of impulse conduction: abnormal automaticity

All parts of the cardiac conduction system demonstrate a spontaneous phase 4 depolarization, and are therefore potential or *latent* pacemakers. Because sinoatrial node (SAN) pacemaking is of the highest frequency (70–80 beats/min), it causes overdrive suppression of pacemaking by the atrioventricular node (AVN) (50–60 beats/min) or Purkinje fibres (30–40 beats/min). However, ischaemia, hypokalaemia, fibre stretch or local catecholamine release may increase automaticity in latent pacemakers, which can then 'escape' from SAN dominance to cause arrhythmias.

Cardiac muscle cells are not normally latent pacemakers. However, even these cells can develop repetitive impulse initiation and cause arrhythmias if the membrane potential is sufficiently depolarized. This usually occurs as a result of underlying cardiac disease, most commonly ischaemia. The threshold at which such **depolarization-induced automaticity** develops is quite variable. Automatic rhythms may demonstrate 'warm up' and 'cool down' phenomena, where the rate gradually accelerates to a constant level and then slows prior to termination of the arrhythmia.

Disorders of impulse conduction: triggered automaticity

Triggered automaticity is caused by **afterdepolarizations**. These are oscillations in the membrane potential which occur during or after repolarization. Oscillations large enough to reach threshold initiate premature action potentials and heart beats. This may occur repeatedly, initiating a sustained arrhythmia (Fig. 46.1a). Afterdepolarization magnitude is influenced by changes in heart rate, catecholamines and parasympathetic withdrawal.

Early afterdepolarizations (EADs) occur during the terminal plateau or repolarization phases of the action potential. They develop more readily in Purkinje fibres than in ventricular or atrial myocytes. EAD can be induced by agents that prolong action potential duration and increase the inward current. For example, drugs such as sotalol, n-acetyl procainamide (a procainamide metabolite) and quinidine block K^+ currents, and can cause EADs and triggered activity by delaying repolarization, especially when the heart rate is slow. The abnormal rhythms induced by such drugs resemble **torsade de pointes**, a type of congenital arrhythmia.

Delayed afterdepolarizations (DADs) occur after repolarization is complete, and are due to excessive increases in cellular $[Ca^{2+}]$. This can be caused by catecholamines, which increase Ca^{2+} influx through the L-type Ca^{2+} channel, and by digitalis glycosides, which increase $[Ca^{2+}]_i$ by a mechanism described in Chapter 45. The **transient inward current** responsible for the oscillation of membrane potential following an increase in $[Ca^{2+}]_i$ appears to be caused by entry of Na^+. The occurrence and magnitude of DADs and the likelihood that they will cause arrhythmias is increased by conditions that enhance the transient inward current. These include longer action potentials, which cause larger increases in $[Ca^{2+}]_i$. Therefore, drugs prolonging action potential duration may trigger DADs, whereas drugs shortening the action potential have the opposite effect. The magnitude of the transient inward current is also influenced by the resting membrane potential, and is maximal when this is approximately $-60\,mV$.

Abnormal impulse conduction: re-entry

Re-entry occurs when an impulse which is delayed in one region of the myocardium re-excites adjacent areas of the myocardium more than once. There are two types of re-entry, anatomical and functional.

Emergence of **anatomical re-entry** requires the presence of several conditions:

1 There must exist an anatomical circuit around which the impulse can circulate. This circuit can utilize parallel conduction pathways such as two Purkinje fibre branches, or the AV node and an accessory atrioventricular conduction pathway (see Chapter 15).
2 Impulse conduction at some point in the circuit should be slow enough to allow the region in front of the impulse to recover from refractoriness.
3 The circuit must also include a zone of unidirectional block where conduction is blocked in one direction while remaining possible in the other.

For example, a re-entrant circuit may develop where two terminal branches (A and B) of a Purkinje fibre enter ventricular muscle (Fig. 46.1b). Under normal conditions, the impulses conducted via either branch excite, and then die out in, the ventricular muscle (Fig. 46.1b(i)). However, if conduction becomes depressed in one branch (see below), it is possible for antero-

grade conduction here to be blocked, while retrograde conduction continues but is slowed (Fig. 46.1b(ii)). In this case, the impulse from A can enter B in a retrograde direction and slowly traverse the zone of unidirectional block. If delayed sufficiently here, the myocardium it re-enters on the other side is no longer refractory, and is re-excited (Fig. 46.1b(iii)). The impulse may then continue to cycle around the triangle formed by the two Purkinje fibres and the ventricular muscle, giving off impulses with each cycle that are conducted throughout the ventricle.

Depressed conduction occurs when the amplitude and slope of phase 0 depolarization are depressed, causing a diminution of axial current flow. *Depressed fast responses* occur when impulses arise in situations where many (but not all) Na^+ channels are inactivated, and therefore unable to open. This can happen if an impulse arises prematurely during the relative refractory period, and also where the resting potential is low (-60 to $-70\,mV$), in which case many channels remain inactivated for an abnormally long time following action potentials. At membrane potential levels positive of $-60\,mV$, Na^+ channels are completely inactivated, but L-type Ca^{2+} channels can still open, resulting in a slowly propagated action potential termed a *slow response*.

Anatomical re-entry may also occur in congenital conditions (**Wolff–Parkinson–White syndrome** and **AV nodal re-entrant tachycardia**) in which the impulse is conducted from the atria to the ventricles via two pathways. These pathways differ with respect to impulse conduction velocity and refractoriness, leading to the development of a functional unidirectional block which allows re-entry to occur (see Chapter 15).

Functional re-entry does not require an anatomically defined circuit, and arises when neighbouring microdomains of the myocardium develop heterogeneous electrical properties. An important example of this is **anisotropic re-entry** (Fig. 46.1c).

Cardiac fibres tend to be arranged in bundles (fascicles). Impulse transmission along the length of a fascicle is rapid, whereas transmission in the transverse direction (i.e. across the fascicle) is slower. This effect, termed **anisotropy**, occurs because gap junctions, which mediate cell-to-cell conduction, are clustered more densely at the ends of the cells.

Following a myocardial infarction, scattered fascicles in the epicardial muscle in the border zone of the infarct may have severely depressed conduction due to a loss of gap junctions, so that their anisotropic properties become exaggerated. In this case, impulse conduction out of the damaged fascicle is blocked at its 'sides' (solid lines, Fig. 46.1c), while impulse conduction in the longitudinal direction remains possible, but is slowed. An impulse entering this fascicle (**1**) is therefore retarded (**2**), so that when it re-enters normal myocardium at the other end of the fascicle, it encounters tissue that is no longer refractory (**3**). This impulse can then propagate in all directions (**4**), abnormally exciting the ventricle, and re-entering the damaged fascicle (**5**) to set up a cycle which continues to re-excite the ventricle at a rapid frequency.

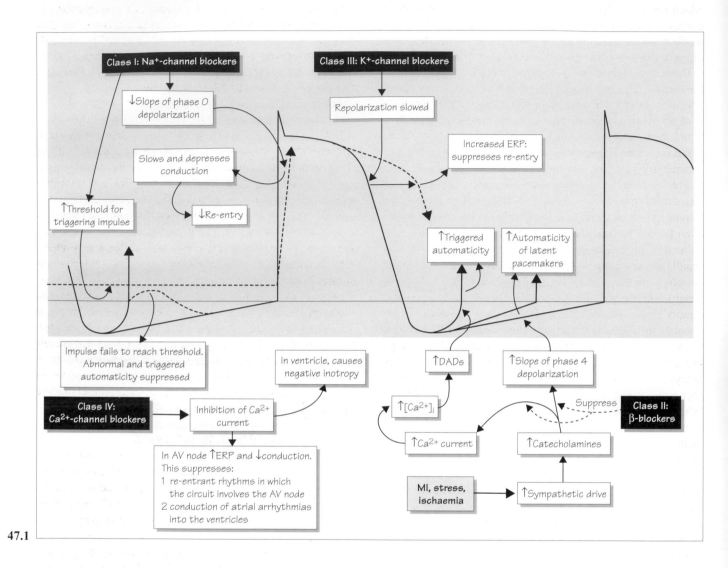

47.1

Most antiarrhythmic drugs, whatever their specific mechanisms, have two actions which allow them to reduce abnormal electrical activity, while having tolerably small effects on normal myocardium:

1 They suppress abnormal (ectopic) pacemakers more than they do the sinoatrial node.

2 They increase the ratio of the effective refractory period to action potential duration: ERP/APD.

Antiarrhythmic drugs have been divided into four classes, based on their cellular mechanisms (Fig. 47.1). However, most antiarrhythmic drugs have properties of more than one of these classes, often because drug metabolites have their own separate antiarrhythmic effects, or because the drugs exist as 50/50 mixtures of two stereoisomers with different actions. This classification system, introduced by Vaughan Williams and Singh, also excludes several drugs, and is of limited use in matching specific

drugs to particular arrhythmias. A more clinically relevant classification scheme is presented in Table 48.1.

Clinical trials over the past 15 years have shown that class I agents do not enhance survival, and in fact are deleterious if used for some purposes (e.g. prevention of ventricular ectopic beats). Conversely, the class III agent amiodarone modestly increases survival, and class II agents (β-blockers) are increasingly seen to be beneficial for virtually the entire spectrum of coronary heart diseases. There is therefore a trend away from the use of class I drugs, towards the use of class II and III drugs. Moreover, the success of radiofrequency catheter ablation in curing some superventricular tachyarrhythmias, as well as the effectiveness of implantable defibrillators in controlling some types of lethal ventricular arrhythmias, is increasingly shifting the emphasis of arrhythmia management towards device-based therapy.

Class I drugs

Class I drugs act primarily by blocking Na^+ channels, an effect which slows and depresses impulse conduction. Depression of conduction can interrupt re-entrant pathways by deepening a unidirectional block, thereby rendering it bidirectional. Class I drugs can also suppress automaticity (Fig. 47.1, upper left).

Because they have a higher affinity for Na^+ channels when they are open and/or inactivated, these drugs bind to Na^+ channels during each action potential and then progressively dissociate following repolarization. Dissociation is slowed in cells in which the resting potential is decreased, and this leads to a deepening of channel blockade in tissue that is depolarized due to ischaemia.

Three subclasses of class I drugs were originally designated based on studies of their effects on the action potential in canine Purkinje fibres, which showed that each class of drug dissociates from the Na^+ channel at different rates. Class IB drugs (**lidocaine, tocainide, mexilitine**) dissociate from the channel very rapidly and almost completely between action potentials. They therefore have little effect in normal myocardium because the steady-state level of drug bound to the channel remains minimal. However, in tissue that is depolarized, or firing at a high frequency, dissociation between impulses is decreased, promoting channel blockade and depression of conduction. These drugs, especially lidocaine, are therefore useful in treating ventricular tachyarrhythmias associated with MI, which mainly originate in myocardium depolarized by ischaemia. Conversely, class IC drugs (**flecainide, propafenone**) dissociate so slowly that they remain bound to channels from one action potential to the next, even at low frequencies of stimulation. This strongly depresses conduction in both normal and depolarized myocardium, which leads to a reduction in cardiac contractility. The intermediate dissociation rate of class IA drugs (**quinidine, procainamide, disopyramide**) causes a lengthening of the effective refractory period. These drugs also have class III activity, which prolongs the action potential.

Class I drugs cause many side effects, not the least of which are several types of arrhythmia. This **proarrhythmic** effect is not surprising, given that depression of conduction and prolongation of the action potential are important prerequisites for arrhythmia development (see Chapter 46).

Class II drugs

β-blockers such as **propranolol, metoprolol, atenolol** and **timolol** form the second class of antiarrhythmics. The rationale for the use of these drugs is that catecholamine elevation associated with MI and heart failure stimulates cardiac β-receptors, and this is thought to cause arrhythmias through multiple mechanisms (Fig. 47.1, lower right; also see Chapter 46). At higher concentrations β-blockers block Na^+ channels, but this action is unlikely to contribute much to their therapeutic effect.

Class III drugs

Class III drugs increase APD and therefore prolong ERP. Re-entry occurs when an impulse is locally delayed, and then re-enters and re-excites adjacent myocardium (see Chapter 46). Drugs which prolong ERP can prevent this re-excitation because the adjacent myocardium is still refractory (inexcitable) at the time when the delayed impulse reaches it. The class III agents **amiodarone, sotalol** and **bretylium** increase APD by inhibiting K^+ channels and slowing repolarization. However, each drug has additional actions, which may be useful.

Amiodarone is effective against many supraventricular and ventricular arrhythmias, probably because it also has class IA, II and IV actions (and blocks α-receptors!). Clinical trials show that amiodarone modestly reduces mortality after MI and in congestive heart failure. However, its long-term use is recommended only if other antiarrhythmic drugs fail, because it has many cumulative adverse effects and must be discontinued in about a third of patients. Hazards include pulmonary fibrosis, hypo- and hyperthyroidism, liver dysfunction, photosensitivity and peripheral neuropathy. Amiodarone also has a very unpredictable and long (4–15 weeks) plasma half-life, which complicates its oral administration. Sotalol is a mixed class II and III drug used for ventricular and supraventricular arrhythmias. Although it causes far fewer side effects than amiodarone, it is more likely to cause torsades de pointes (see Chapter 46). **Dofetilide, ibutilide** and **azimilide** are newer drugs that are relatively selective for the voltage-gated K^+ channels involved in repolarization. These drugs are used to terminate atrial flutter and fibrillation. They can also cause torsades de pointes in some patients, although azimilide is less apt to do so.

Class IV drugs, adenosine and digoxin

Class IV drugs (**verapamil, diltiazem**) exert their antiarrhythmic effects on the atrioventricular node (AVN) by blocking L-type Ca^{2+} channels. These channels mediate the AVN action potential, and their blockade therefore slows AVN depolarization and conduction, and also increases the refractory period. Ca^{2+}-channel blockade is use dependent, and AV block is enhanced by cell depolarization and high-frequency firing. These drugs are used to treat supraventricular tachycardias. They suppress AV nodal re-entrant rhythms by depressing conduction. They can slow the ventricular rate in atrial flutter and fibrillation by preventing a proportion of atrial impulses from being conducted through the AVN. Negative inotropy can occur due to L-type channel inhibition, especially if left ventricular function is impaired. Negative inotropic and chronotropic effects are exacerbated by coadministration of β-blockers.

Adenosine, an endogenous nucleoside (see Chapter 22), acts on myocardial A_1-receptors, suppressing the Ca^{2+} current and enhancing K^+ currents. These effects depress AV nodal conduction. Adenosine is the drug of choice for rapid termination of many supraventricular tachycardias. It commonly causes transient flushing and breathlessness. **Digoxin** slows AV conduction by stimulating the vagus and is used to slow atrial fibrillation and other supraventricular tachycardias, especially in patients with heart failure (see Chapter 45).

48 Specific arrhythmias

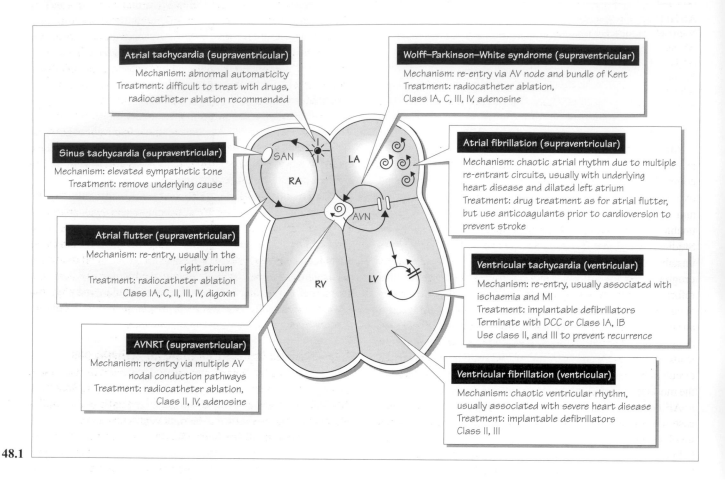

48.1

Figure 48.1 summarizes the mechanisms and treatments for common arrhythmias. All of these cause tachycardia; bradyarrhythmias are described in Chapter 15.

Supraventricular tachycardias (SVTs)

Supraventricular tachycardias are abnormalities in the timing or sequence of cardiac depolarization, originating at or above the atrioventricular node, which result in a heart rate of > 100 beats/min. Most of these are troublesome rather than life threatening. Common symptoms include lightheadedness, palpitations and shortness of breath. Rarely, sudden death can occur.

Sinus tachycardia (100–200 beats/min), the most common SVT, occurs when physiological (exercise) or pathological (phaeochromocytoma, congestive heart failure, thyrotoxicosis) stimuli elevate the sympathetic tone and accelerate SA nodal pacemaking. Sinus tachycardia generally starts and stops gradually. Treatment involves removing the underlying cause.

Atrial tachycardia is frequently caused by an abnormal (ectopic) pacemaker, and can occur in either atrium. Some atrial tachycardias are re-entrant in nature, frequently following sur-

gery that involves incision into the atrium. The onset and offset of the tachycardia may be sudden or gradual.

Atrial flutter results from re-entry in an atrium (usually the right), with an area of slowed conduction near the orifice of the inferior vena cava and a circuit involving the whole atrium. The atrial rate is typically 300 beats/min, with a ventricular rate that is 150 (2 : 1), 100 (3 : 1) or 75 (4 : 1) per minute depending on AVN conduction. Both atrial flutter and atrial fibrillation (see below) are typically seen in patients with underlying cardiac disease, often associated with atrial dilatation. These conditions are particularly common in older hypertensives, and may also be caused by acute pulmonary thromboembolism or thyrotoxicosis. Both conditions can also develop paroxysmally in patients without underlying heart disease. Attempts to **cardiovert** (restore normal sinus rhythm) atrial flutter with class IA drugs may cause severe ventricular tachycardia and sudden death by establishing 1 : 1 AV nodal conduction. This occurs because these drugs suppress vagal firing, thereby increasing AV nodal conduction. This hazard is avoided by preadministering a drug that suppresses AVN conduction (e.g. a β-blocker).

Table 48.1 Classification of antiarrhythmic drugs based on site(s) of action

Atria: Dofetilide, ibutelide
Ventricles: Lidocaine, mexilitine, tocainide
AV node: Adenosine, β-blockers, verapamil, diltiazem, digoxin
Atria and ventricles, AV accessory pathways: Amiodarone, flecainide, propafenone, procainamide, disopyramide, quinidine, sotalol

Atrial fibrillation (AF) is a chaotic atrial rhythm resulting in an atrial rate of 350–600 beats/min and a lack of effective atrial contraction. AF is very common, occurring in ~10% of people over the age of 75. The ventricular rate is 'irregularly irregular' and is typically less than 200 beats/min, because the AVN is unable to conduct most of the atrial impulses impinging upon it. Studies suggest that this arrhythmia is caused by five to seven unstable re-entrant circuits with very short cycle lengths, which progress across the atrium, temporarily disappearing and then reforming. Palpitations, dyspnoea, presyncope or syncope may occur due to the increased ventricular rate or the absence of atrial systolic filling. Thrombi may form in the left atrial cavity or appendage because the lack of coordinated atrial contraction leads to stasis of blood. These can then embolize to the systemic circulation, particularly the brain and limbs, so that fibrillation is the most important cause of stroke in the elderly.

AF can occur episodically, or can be permanent, in which case it is more difficult to control. Pharmacological treatment involves restoring normal sinus rhythm, often with amiodarone ('rhythm control'). Alternatively, a class IV or other agent is used to suppress AV conduction, thereby reducing the frequency of impulses which reach and excite the ventricles ('rate control').

Wolff–Parkinson–White syndrome and **atrioventricular re-entrant tachycardias** are re-entrant tachycardias which depend on the presence of a congenital accessory conduction pathway between atria and ventricles, as described in Chapter 15.

Ventricular arrhythmias

Ventricular tachycardia (VT) originates in the ventricles, and is defined as four or more successive ventricular ectopic beats. The rate, frequency of recurrence and duration of VT can vary widely between individuals, as can its consequences. In some, it may cause haemodynamic collapse or degenerate into ventricular fibrillation, but in other people it may be of little consequence.

The ECG demonstrates a rapid, broad complex rhythm, with a bizarre QRS complex. Normal atrial activation may continue to be driven by the SA node, or the abnormal ventricular pacemaker may cause atrial tachycardia via impulses moving 'backwards' through the AV node. VT can be either **monomorphic**, in which case the QRS complexes all have a similar configuration, or **polymorphic**, where the QRS complexes progressively wax and wane in amplitude, appearing to twist around the baseline. **Torsade de pointes** is a type of polymorphic VT in which

brief episodes of tachycardia are superimposed upon intervals of bradycardia with a prolonged QT interval.

VT is usually associated with structural heart disease, in which case it has a poor prognosis, with 50% mortality at 2 years. It very often results from micro re-entrant circuits occurring in the border zone of myocardial infarcts (see Chapter 46), and these rhythms may be initiated by ventricular ectopic beats caused by an automatic or triggered automatic mechanism. It is also associated with cardiomyopathy, and valvular and congenital heart disease. VT is uncommon in structurally normal hearts, but specific varieties are recognized, including right ventricular ouflow tract tachycardia and fascicular tachycardia. These have a good prognosis, and can usually be treated with radiofrequency catheter ablation.

Ventricular fibrillation (VF) is a chaotic ventricular rhythm causing an immediate loss of cardiac output and death unless the patient is resuscitated. VF may follow episodes of VT or acute ischaemia, and frequently occurs during MI. It is the main cause of sudden death, which is responsible for ~10% of all mortality. VF is generally associated with severe underlying heart disease, including ischaemic heart disease and cardiomyopathy, but occurs occasionally in a normal heart (idiopathic VF). Following one event, there is a high recurrence rate.

Nonpharmacological treatment for arrhythmias

Direct current (DC) cardioversion allows rapid cardioversion of VF and haemodynamically unstable SVT and VT. Shocks of 50–360 J are delivered to the anaesthetized patient via paddles placed over the sternum and the right ventricular apex.

In **radiofrequency catheter ablation** the accessory pathways or focally automatic myocardium causing certain tachyarrhythmias are ablated by focal heating delivered via a catheter. The catheter is placed transvenously and the tip is located at the surface of the endocardium at the site of the abnormality. Radiofrequency energy is delivered to the catheter tip, and dissipated to a large indifferent plate, usually over the back. The tip temperature is set to 60–65°C, resulting in a lesion 8–10 mm in diameter and of a similar depth. This extremely safe technique is curative in > 90% of certain supraventricular arrhythmias.

Implantable defibrillators consist of a generator connected to electrodes placed transvenously in the heart and superior vena cava. A sensing circuit detects arrhythmias, which are classified as tachycardia or fibrillation on the basis of rate. The treatment algorithm is either as burst pacing, which can terminate VT with a high degree of success, or by the delivery of a shock at up to 40 J, which can cardiovert VT and VF. Shock delivery is between an electrode in the right ventricle and another in the superior vena cava or to the body of the generator (active can). Refinements in detection allow the distinction of supraventricular and ventricular arrhythmias, so that several tiers of progressively more aggressive therapy can be set up. The AVID study reported in 1997 that in patients with malignant ventricular arrhythmia, this approach improved survival by 31% over 3 years compared to antiarrhythmic drug therapy (mainly amiodarone).

49 Diseases of the aortic valve

(a) Aortic stenosis

Signs
- Low volume slow rising pulse
- Heaving apex
- Ejection systolic murmur

Pathophysiology
- Aortic valve narrowing
- Pressure overload of LV
- LV hypertrophy
- Turbulent ejection of blood across aortic valve

Aorta
LV

LV pressure
Gradient
Aortic pressure
Pressure (mmHg)
200
100
0

Ejection systolic murmur
S_1 Ec S_2

Causes of aortic valve stenosis
Congenital
Rheumatic heart disease
Acquired calcification and fibrosis of valve or chordae tendineae with age

(b) Aortic regurgitation

Signs
- Collapsing pulse
- Displaced heaving apex
- Diastolic murmur

Pathophysiology
- Aortic valve leaking
- Ventricular enlargement (due to forward flow and regurgitant flow held in ventricle)
- Ventricular hypertrophy
- Diastolic leaking back of blood from aorta
- Jet may cause vibration of anterior leaflet of mitral valve
- Austin–Flint murmurs + early closure of mitral valve

S_1 S_2

Systolic murmur due to increased flow over aortic valve

Early diastolic regurgitant murmur

Causes of aortic valve regurgitation

Rheumatic heart disease	Dilation of aortic root:
Infective endocarditis	age-associated degeneration
Congenital	Marfan's syndrome
Inflammatory disease	aortic dissection
systemic lupus erythematosus	
rheumatoid arthritis ankylosing	Systemic diseases:
spondylitis	Syphilis
	Ulcerative colitis
	Behçet's disease
	Giant cell arteritis

49.1

The **aortic valve** is normally tricuspid and separates the left ventricle (LV) from the aorta. Impaired aortic valve opening (**aortic stenosis**, AS) impedes outflow of blood and imposes a pressure load on the LV. Deficient valve closure (**aortic regurgitation**, AR, *incompetence*) allows blood to flow back from the aorta, and imposes a volume load on the LV.

Aortic stenosis
Causes
Acquired calcific aortic stenosis is the most common cause. Calcium deposits occur at the base of the cusp, without involvement of the commissures. This is most likely related to pro-

longed mechanical stress, and is more common in people with congenital bicuspid valves. About 50% of patients < 70 years old with significant AS have bicuspid valves, whereas most old patients with AS have tricuspid valves.

Rheumatic: AS as a result of rheumatic heart disease is unusual without coexisting mitral valve disease. Male sex, diabetes and hypercholesterolaemia are also risk factors for AS.

Congenital: A **unicuspid aortic valve** is usually fatal within 1 year from birth. **Bicuspid** aortic valves develop progressive fusion of the commissures, and symptoms usually present after 40 years. Infants with atherosclerosis due to lipid disorders may develop AS in conjunction with **coronary artery disease** (CAD).

Pathophysiology

A slow reduction of aortic valve area causes **left ventricular hypertrophy** and eventual myocardial dysfunction, arrhythmias, and **left heart failure** (see Chapter 44). 'Critical' AS occurs with > 75% reduction of valve area to < 0.5 cm²/m² body surface area, and a > 50 mmHg gradient between peak systolic LV and aortic pressure at a normal cardiac output. With worsening AS, cardiac output cannot increase adequately during exercise and eventually becomes insufficient at rest. At this point the LV dilates, and left ventricular end-diastolic pressure (EDP) increases to the point where overt LV failure ensues.

Clinical features

Patients present usually between the ages of 50 and 70 years, most commonly with **angina** (50% have concurrent CAD). Angina is due to the increased oxygen needs of the hypertrophied LV and inadequate cardiac output during exercise. Exercise tolerance is decreased, and if brain bloodflow is insufficient patients may develop **exercise-associated syncope**. Once patients with AS develop angina, syncope or LV failure, their median survival is < 3 years.

Patients with mild AS have a normal blood pressure and pulse. In moderate to severe AS there is a slow-rising, low-volume pulse that may demonstrate a **thrill** (vibration) and decreased pulse pressure. Auscultation reveals a normal S_1, a single S_2 because of an absent aortic component, a S_4, and a harsh late **systolic murmur**, preceded by an ejection click (Ec) (see Fig. 49.1a and Chapter 13), heard best in the right second intercostal space and transmitted to the carotids and apex. It is louder with squatting and softer with standing or during the **Valsalva manoeuvre** (forced expiration against a closed glottis). With worsening AS and a fall in cardiac output, the murmur may become softer (**silent AS**).

Investigations

The ECG shows LV hypertrophy with strain (depressed ST, inverted T), and left atrial delay. Atrial fibrillation and ventricular arrhythmias are often seen when LV function has deteriorated. Echocardiography shows reduced valve opening and calcification of cusps, and allows calculation of valve area. Doppler imaging allows calculation of the pressure gradient between the LV and aorta.

Management

It is important that systemic hypotension and arterial vasodilatation be avoided. β-adrenergic blockers and other negative inotropic agents should thus not be used. Once symptoms develop, cardiac catheterization with **coronary angiography** must be performed prior to valve replacement, and coronary artery bypass performed if significant CAD is present. Several types of mechanical valve are available, including those of a 'ball and cage' variety or tilting disc. These will always require **anticoagulant therapy**. Valves can also be obtained from pigs or human cadavers and these have the advantage that anticoagulants are not generally required. **Balloon valvuloplasty** can be performed in children with noncalcified valves, but is of little value in adults.

Aortic regurgitation
Causes

Causes of aortic regurgitation (AR) include **rheumatic disease**, where fibrous retraction of the valve cusps prevents apposition, **infective endocarditis** causing valve damage, and **congenital malformations** (e.g. bicuspid valve) (see Fig. 49.1, right).

Pathophysiology

AR imposes a volume load on the LV because of flow back into the ventricle. **Acute AR** (trauma, infective endocarditis, aortic dissection) is usually catastrophic. Here the LV cannot accommodate the acute increase in volume and LVEDP rises. The early increase in LVEDP causes premature closure of the mitral valve and inadequate forward LV filling, resulting in cardiovascular collapse and acute respiratory failure.

In **chronic AR**, volume load and LVEDP increase gradually, and **LV hypertrophy** allows adequate output to be maintained. As the aortic valve never completely closes, there is no LV isovolumetric relaxation phase (see Chapter 13) and the pulse pressure is wide.

Clinical features

Patients usually do not present with symptoms until LV failure develops. Signs include a wide pulse pressure (caused by reduction in diastolic pressure) and a **collapsing pulse** (Chapter 13). This may occasionally cause visible nail bed pulsation and pulsatile head bobbing. The LV apex is displaced laterally and is hyperdynamic. Auscultation reveals a high-pitched **early diastolic murmur** at the left sternal border, and a **systolic flow murmur** across the aortic valve. A low-frequency **rumbling late diastolic murmur** at the apex (**Austin–Flint murmur**) may be caused by premature closing of the mitral valve.

Investigations

Echocardiography can determine the aetiology and severity of AR by imaging the valve leaflets and LV dimensions, aortic root diameter, and diastolic closure or fluttering of the mitral valve. Doppler imaging quantifies the amount of regurgitation.

Management

Acute severe AR requires urgent valve replacement. Chronic AR has a generally good prognosis until symptoms develop. Patients with moderate AR should be followed with serial echocardiography. Valve replacement should be considered in patients with symptoms, or in asymptomatic patients with worsening LV dimensions, LV function, or aortic root diameter. Valve replacement is similar to that for aortic stenosis, except that replacement of the aortic root may also be required in patients with a severely dilated ascending aorta.

Diseases of the mitral valve

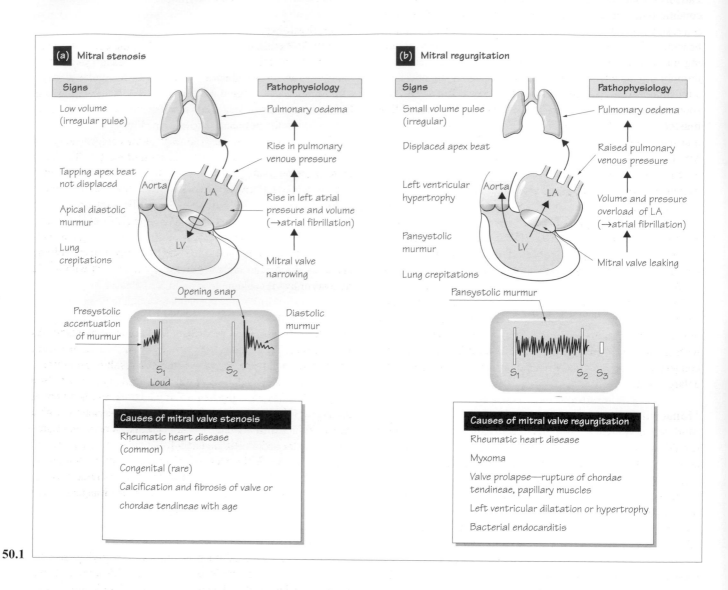

50.1

The **mitral valve** is normally bicuspid and separates the left atrium (LA) and left ventricle (LV). The valve may narrow (**mitral stenosis**) or leak (**mitral regurgitation**).

Mitral stenosis
Causes
Mitral stenosis (MS) is usually due to prior episodes of acute **rheumatic fever**. This causes thickening and fusion of the mitral **commissures**, **cusps**, or **chordae tendineae**, making the cusps less flexible and narrowing the orifice. Symptoms from MS usually develop > 10 years after the acute attack, which patients may not recall. The normal area of a mitral valve is 6 cm²; critical MS occurs when this area falls to 1 cm².

Pathophysiology
Mitral stenosis prevents the free flow of blood from the LA to the LV, and slows ventricular filling during diastole. The left atrial pressure rises to maintain cardiac output, and there is **atrial hypertrophy** and **dilatation**. The elevated left atrial pressure causes pulmonary congestion and can result in **pulmonary hypertension** and **oedema**, and **right heart failure** (see Chapter 44). Patients with MS rely on atrial systole for ventricular filling, and **atrial fibrillation** (caused by atrial enlargement) significantly reduces cardiac output. The fibrillating atrium is liable to develop **thrombi** that may be **embolized** (dislodge and move freely in the blood) causing stroke. The LV is usually normal in MS, but may be abnormal due to either chronic underfeeding of the LV or rheumatic scarring.

Clinical features

Patients present in their 20–30s with **dyspnoea** on exertion or conditions that raise cardiac output (e.g. fever, pregnancy). This is a result of **pulmonary congestion**, which causes the lungs to become stiffer. Patients may present with **haemoptysis** (coughing up of blood), **palpitations** or **stroke** (via embolization of thrombi). Symptoms may be precipitated by arrhythmias such as atrial fibrillation. Auscultation reveals an **opening snap** (OS) soon after S_2 that is heard best at the apex, and by a **rumbling diastolic murmur** leading to a loud S_1. The duration of the murmur is related to the severity of the MS. It is brief in mild MS and **holodiastolic** (*pandiastolic*, i.e. over the whole diastolic period) in severe MS. Patients in sinus rhythm may have **presystolic accentuation** of the murmur due to atrial contraction, and a large venous 'a' wave (see Chapter 13). If the mitral valve is completely immobile there may be no OS or a loud S_1. As MS becomes more severe, there will be a less prominent arterial pulse, **lung crackles** (*crepitations*; audible crackles because of fluid in the lungs), and elevation of the **jugular venous pressure**.

The ECG may show only LA enlargement, although many patients are in atrial fibrillation. The chest radiograph may show left atrial enlargement with normal left ventricular size, but with increasing severity of MS there may be pulmonary vascular congestion, enlarged pulmonary arteries, and right ventricular enlargement.

Management

Mild MS may require little treatment, although management should include avoidance of **anaemia** and **tachyarrhythmias** as these may precipitate decompensation and cardiac failure (see Chapter 44). Prophylactic antibiotics for **endocarditis** should be administered before invasive procedures and patients in atrial fibrillation should receive **anticoagulation** to decrease the occurrence of stroke. Patients with MS can remain minimally symptomatic for many years, but deteriorate quickly once symptoms begin to worsen. Therefore, **valve replacement** with a mechanical valve, **valvotomy** (surgical separation of commissures) or **balloon valvuloplasty** (use of a balloon catheter to force open cusps) should be performed in moderately symptomatic patients with a mitral valve area < 1.7 cm².

Mitral regurgitation

Causes

Acute mitral regurgitation (MR) is usually a result of **bacterial endocarditis, ruptured chordae tendineae**, or ischaemic **papillary muscle rupture**. Chronic MR is now most likely to arise from **myxomatous degeneration** of the mitral leaflets or **valve prolapse** (reversal into atrium). Chronic MR may also develop in any disease causing LV dilatation, so preventing apposition (coming together) of the mitral leaflets, or because of ischaemic dysfunction of the papillary muscles.

Pathophysiology

In **acute MR** the LV ejects blood back into the LA, imposing a sudden volume load on the LA during ventricular systole. Left atrial pressure rises suddenly and this is rapidly followed by a rise in pulmonary venous pressure and capillary pressure. **Pulmonary oedema** ensues as a result of alteration of haemodynamics across the pulmonary vascular bed.

Chronic MR is sufficiently slow to allow compensatory LV dilatation and hypertrophy, and dilatation of the LA. The latter protects the pulmonary circulation from the effects of the regurgitant volume. MR imposes a diastolic volume load on the LV that causes dilatation, because each systolic stroke volume is composed of a portion that enters the aorta (LV output) and an ineffective portion that re-enters the LA (LV regurgitant volume) and adds to the venous return. The regurgitant volume increases when LV emptying is impaired, such as with aortic stenosis or hypertension.

Clinical features

Patients with mild chronic MR are usually asymptomatic. As MR worsens, patients develop **fatigue, dyspnoea on exertion, orthopnoea** and **pulmonary oedema** as a result of progressive LV failure and elevation of pulmonary capillary pressure (see Chapter 44). The development of atrial fibrillation is common because of dilatation of the LA. Chronic MR is associated with a **holosystolic** murmur which is heard best at the apex, with transmission to the axilla and the left infrascapular region. S_1 is soft and S_2 is split widely because of an early aortic component. Echocardiography can detect a prolapsing or rheumatic valve, and determine LV size and function. Doppler imaging of the regurgitant jet can assess the severity of MR.

Management

Management is focused on promoting LV emptying into the aorta. Reduction of afterload with **ACE inhibitors** is beneficial (see Chapter 45). Patients with atrial fibrillation receive **anticoagulants** to prevent stroke. A prolapsing valve may sometimes be repaired. Dilatation of the mitral valve ring may be corrected by implantation of an artificial ring. Rheumatic valves and those damaged by endocarditis often need replacement with an artificial valve. Valve replacement is best performed prior to the development of LV dysfunction or chronic pulmonary hypertension, and should always be performed in patients with symptomatic MR despite medical therapy. The risks of surgery are higher in acute MR; however, valve replacement should be performed in patients with uncontrollable heart failure or end-organ failure, even in cases of acute infective endocarditis.

51 Congenital heart disease

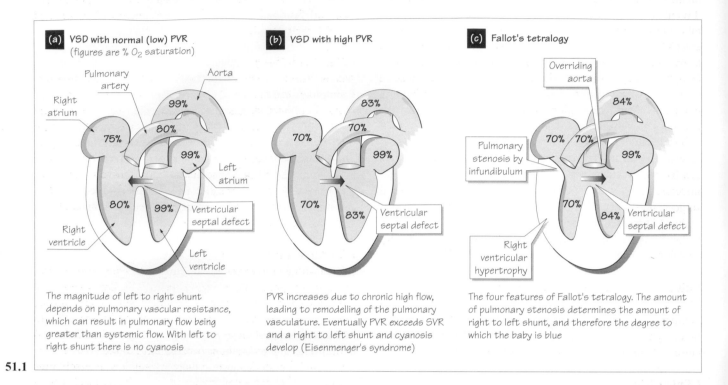

(a) VSD with normal (low) PVR
(figures are % O₂ saturation)

Pulmonary artery — Aorta
Right atrium
99%
80%
75%
99%
Left atrium
80%
99%
Ventricular septal defect
Right ventricle
Left ventricle

The magnitude of left to right shunt depends on pulmonary vascular resistance, which can result in pulmonary flow being greater than systemic flow. With left to right shunt there is no cyanosis

(b) VSD with high PVR

83%
70%
70%
99%
70%
83%
Ventricular septal defect

PVR increases due to chronic high flow, leading to remodelling of the pulmonary vasculature. Eventually PVR exceeds SVR and a right to left shunt and cyanosis develop (Eisenmenger's syndrome)

(c) Fallot's tetralogy

Overriding aorta
84%
Pulmonary stenosis by infundibulum
70% 70%
99%
70%
84%
Ventricular septal defect
Right ventricular hypertrophy

The four features of Fallot's tetralogy. The amount of pulmonary stenosis determines the amount of right to left shunt, and therefore the degree to which the baby is blue

51.1

Definition
Congenital heart diseases (CHDs) are abnormalities of cardiac structure that are present from birth. They result from abnormalities in cardiac development occurring between 3 and 8 weeks of gestation.

Incidence
The incidence of CHD is ~1% of live births, not including congenital valve disorders such as mitral prolapse or bicuspid aortic valve. Many spontaneous abortions or stillborns have cardiac malformations, or chromosomal abnormalities associated with structural heart defects. Maternal factors such as **rubella infection**, alcohol abuse and some medications are associated with CHD.

Physiology
In the normal fetal circulation (see Chapter 25) blood crosses the **foramen ovale** from the right to the left atrium. Most of the blood ejected by the right ventricle enters the aorta via the **ductus arteriosus**, because pulmonary vascular resistance (PVR) is higher than systemic vascular resistance (SVR). After birth, PVR falls to one-tenth of SVR, allowing bloodflow from the right ventricle through the lungs. Closure of the foramen ovale and ductus arteriosus establishes the adult circulations in series.

Clinical features
CHDs normally present in infancy with either **congestive heart failure** or **central cyanosis**. Congestive heart failure in an infant is usually due to a left to right shunt, such as a **ventricular septal defect** or a **patent ductus arteriosus** (PDA), or as a result of aortic coarctation or stenosis. Infants with congestive heart failure fail to thrive, and demonstrate symptoms similar to those in adults (see Chapter 44). **Central cyanosis**, blueness of the trunk and mucous membranes, is due to > 3–5 g/dl of deoxygenated haemoglobin in the arterial circulation. Central cyanosis may result from severe pulmonary disease, and intrapulmonary right to left shunt (arteriovenous malformation, AVM) or extrapulmonary right to left shunting. It is characteristic of **transposition of the great vessels** and **tetralogy of Fallot**.

Ventricular septal defect
This is the most common CHD (0.2% births), and may occur in isolation or with other abnormalities. Flow across the defect is determined by the relationship between the resistances of the pulmonary and systemic circulations. *In utero*, when PVR > SVR, most blood exits the left ventricle via the aorta. However, after birth PVR < SVR, and blood is shunted from the left to the right ventricle, and into the pulmonary artery (Fig. 51.1a). The magnitude of the shunt is related to the size of the defect as well as the relative sizes of PVR and SVR.

Clinical features

Ventricular septal defects (VSDs) should be suspected in an infant who fails to gain weight, and has frequent respiratory difficulties or infections. The VSD is diagnosed by a harsh systolic murmur at the left sternal border. In young children a moderate VSD may cause exercise limitation or fatigue, an enlarged heart, and biventricular hypertrophy. Echocardiography with Doppler imaging allows estimation of the size and location of the VSD. Shunting of blood from the left ventricle into the pulmonary circulation leads to pulmonary hypertension, which if persistent causes irreversible **pulmonary vascular remodelling**. Once PVR exceeds SVR the direction of the shunt reverses and cyanosis develops (Fig. 51.1b; **Eisenmenger's syndrome**). At this point surgical correction is not possible, and therefore infants with a significant VSD benefit from early surgery. In the case of smaller VSDs, 50% close spontaneously within 3–4 years. Children with VSDs have an increased risk of endocarditis and should receive prophylactic antibiotics before dental procedures.

Patent (or persistent) ductus arteriosus

PDA may arise because the duct does not close properly due to malformations, and is more common in females. The malformation may be caused by maternal rubella. The duct may also not close in premature babies due to immaturity.

Clinical features

Frequently PDA is not diagnosed immediately after birth, and then only after development of heart failure or infective endocarditis. A loud murmur is characteristically heard in both systole and diastole. The left atrium and ventricle are enlarged. Treatment should be initiated as soon as possible to prevent development of full heart failure. Ligation of the ductus arteriosus is a safe procedure, but must be performed within 5 years of birth. In some cases treatment with indomethacin, a cyclooxygenase inhibitor, to reduce PGE_1 is sufficient to promote closure on its own.

Transposition of the great arteries

Transposition of the great arteries occurs when the left ventricle empties into the pulmonary artery and the right ventricle empties into the aorta. This may be associated with VSD, atrial septal defect (ASD) or PDA. The transposition results in two parallel circulations, where deoxygenated systemic venous blood is returned to the body and oxygenated pulmonary venous blood returns to the lungs. This causes severe central cyanosis. Unless corrected, this defect is fatal in one-third of cases within 2 weeks and in 90% of cases within a year. Surgical correction involves an arterial switch where the great vessels are transected and connected to their appropriate ventricles. Prior to surgery

infants can be stabilized by the creation of an ASD with a catheter, which allows mixing of blood in the atria and oxygenation of systemic blood. Administration of PGE_1 delays closure of the ductus arteriosus and allows further access of oxygenated blood to the systemic circulation.

Fallot's tetralogy

This is the most common cyanotic CHD found in children surviving to 1 year (Fig. 51.1c). It consists of a VSD, pulmonary stenosis, an overriding aorta (positioning of the aorta over the VSD) and right ventricular hypertrophy. These lead to a high right ventricular pressure and right to left shunt. The degree of cyanosis depends on the pulmonary stenosis, which is usually a combination of infundibular stenosis and obstruction of the pulmonary valve. The subvalvular stenosis is caused by misalignment of the infundibular septum; when the latter contracts it may exacerbate the stenosis.

Clinical features

Infants with Fallot's tetralogy are slow to develop, and may present with dyspnoea, fatigue and hypoxic episodes (**Fallot's or tetralogy spells**), characterized by rapidly worsening cyanosis, progressing to limpness, stroke and loss of consciousness. There is usually a palpable RV impulse and a thrill at the left sternal border. There is no pulmonary component to the second heart sound, and a systolic ejection murmur which is inversely proportional to the degree of pulmonary stenosis. Surgical correction of the VSD and ventricular obstruction is performed in infancy and has < 5% mortality.

Atrial septal defects

These defects usually go unrecognized until adulthood. They generally involve the mid-septum in the ostium secundum and are distinct from a patent foramen ovale. The left to right shunt increases pulmonary bloodflow, which if sustained into adulthood leads to pulmonary vascular remodelling and fixed pulmonary hypertension. Adults with ASDs may also present with atrial arrhythmias or left ventricular failure. Once severe pulmonary hypertension develops, there may be reversal of the left to right shunt, and cyanosis due to a right to left shunt.

Clinical features

There is normally a pulmonary ejection murmur, a wide fixed split S_2, and elevated jugular venous pressure. As pulmonary hypertension worsens, the murmur becomes softer and the S_2 becomes louder. If discovered early, ASDs with significant left to right shunts should be repaired to prevent the development of irreversible pulmonary hypertension. Once a right to left shunt has developed, surgical repair of an ASD is not performed.

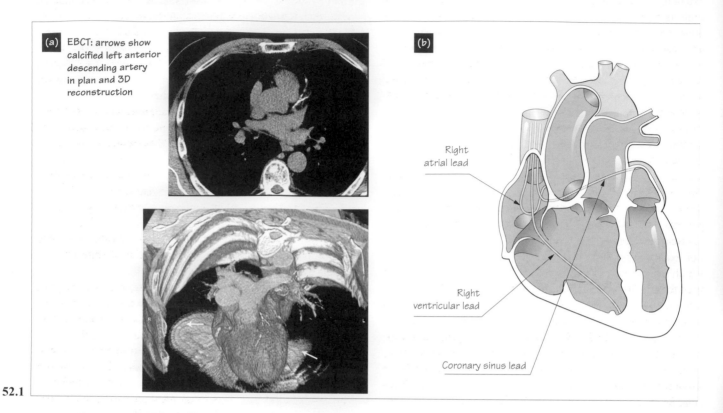

(a) EBCT: arrows show calcified left anterior descending artery in plan and 3D reconstruction

(b)

Right atrial lead

Right ventricular lead

Coronary sinus lead

52.1

The integration of technology, basic science and clinical science have translated into rapid advances in the diagnosis and treatment of cardiovascular diseases.

Cardiovascular risk and its management

Over the past decade, there has been an ever-increasing emphasis placed on the **comprehensive management of cardiovascular risk**. According to the World Health Organization, 75% of the approximately 32 million deaths from heart attacks and stroke that occur worldwide each year can be attributed to hypertension, diabetes, obesity and hyperlidaemias, which are themselves associated with smoking, an unhealthy diet and physical inactivity. It is increasingly realized that the benefits of treating any one individual risk factor, for example hypertension, are greatly enhanced if other risk factors are simultaneously targeted. Moreover, new recommendations make it clear that both the threshold at which it becomes appropriate to treat each risk factor, and the target level to which it should be reduced, need to be made progressively lower if other risk factors are present (see for example the hierarchy of risk-related LDL cholesterol targets listed in Chapter 33).

Although it has long been appreciated that **inflammation** is important in the pathogenesis of atherosclerosis, it is only recently that plasma markers of inflammation have become important tools in the assessment of cardiovascular risk.

Activated macrophages in the atherosclerotic plaque release chemotactic factors, cytokines and growth factors that promote plaque formation and instability. Elevated levels of the acute phase reactant, **C-reactive protein (CRP)**, are associated with cardiovascular disease, myocardial infarction and stroke. CRP inhibits the production of nitric oxide and induces the production of proinflammatory mediators IL-6 and monocyte chemoattractant protein-1 (MCP-1). Elevated CRP levels predict cardiovascular disease in healthy men and women, and may add information to classic cardiovascular risk factors for risk stratification. Recent data show that statin drugs may reduce cardiovascular risk in patients with elevated CRP, and suggest that CRP levels may predict which patients are especially likely to benefit from these drugs. It is not known, however, whether drug therapy to lower CRP levels *per se* will reduced cardiovascular risk. **Lipoprotein-associated phospholipase A$_2$ (Lp-APA$_2$)** may also be a marker of inflammation associated with cardiovascular disease.

Another important concept which has recently emerged is that of the **acute coronary syndromes**. These syndromes, which include **unstable angina (UA)**, **non-ST segment myocardial infarction (NSTEMI)** and **ST segment myocardial infarction (STEMI)**, form a continuous and overlapping spectrum of progressively more serious conditions which are all thought to be initiated by the same key event: formation of a coronary thrombus (see Chapters 38, 41, 42). Depending on various factors, including the location of the thrombus, the extent to which endogenous fibrinolytic mechanisms are able to limit its extent or lifetime, the pre-existing state of the myocardium, and the involvement of other mechanisms such as coronary vasoconstriction, the resulting cardiac ischaemia may be relatively mild and transient or fatally damaging. The crucial difference between UA/NSTEMI and STEMI is that only the latter is appropriately treated with thrombolytics. The main difference between UA and NSTEMI/STEMI is that measurable cardiac necrosis, as seen by the elevation of plasma markers of cardiac cell death, is not seen in the former.

The occurrence of either UA or NSTEMI in a patient indicates a very high risk that coronary thrombosis will recur. However, this risk varies very considerably between different people, therefore **risk stratification** is essential to identify patients who will benefit from early invasive procedures (i.e. revascularization) or who are at high risk of subsequent events. For example, the **TIMI risk score** is a simple scoring system which illustrates how the presence of various factors can be used for rapid risk assessment of patients with UA/NSTEMI. It arose from an analysis of clinical characteristics and outcomes in patients who participated in the Thrombolysis in Myocardial Infarction IIb and ESSENCE trials. The investigators analysed which risk factors, when found at admission to the hospital, were best able to predict whether patients would die, suffer an MI or require urgent revascularization, within 14 days of admission. Seven risk factors were found. These were: age more than 65 years, the presence of three or more risk factors for coronary artery disease, prior presence of a coronary stenosis of $\geq 50\%$, ST segment deviation on ECG, two episodes of angina within the last 24 h, use of aspirin within the last week, and elevated markers of cardiac necrosis. The presence of each factor contributes one point to the overall score. The analysis found, for example, that patients with 0–1 of these risk factors had a 5% chance of suffering one of the outcomes, while 41% of patients with 6–7 factors present went on to experience one of the outcomes within the 14-day period specified. This and other similar risk-predicting schemes are of increasing importance in matching the nature and intensity of treatments to patient risk in order to best utilize the limited financial resources available to health care systems worldwide.

New techniques
Electron beam ('ultrafast') CT (EBCT) allows highly detailed imaging of the heart and coronary anatomy (Fig. 52.1a). EBCT demonstrates coronary calcification that is correlated with atherosclerosis. Quantification of coronary calcium on EBCT allows calculation of a **calcium score**. A low calcium score is associated with a low risk of coronary artery disease. Moderate

to high calcium scores can combine with other noninvasive information for risk stratification. Blacks seem to have lower calcium scores than whites with similar cardiac risk factors. EBCT with intravenous contrast may create images comparable to conventional coronary angiography. Cardiac MRI is currently utilized to demonstrate aortic dissection, pericardial disease, masses and congenital abnormalities. Further refinements in resolution, gating and acquisition time may allow noninvasive coronary angiography and detection of myocardial metabolic ischemia.

Patients with **heart failure** and an **intraventricular conduction delay** have more symptoms and worse outcomes than patients with a normal QRS duration. **Ventricular resynchronization therapy** utilizes biventricular pacing to improve cardiac function. Resynchonization is achieved by placing pacemaker wires in the right atrium, right ventricle and left ventricular free wall (Fig. 52.1b). Resynchonization may result in improved left ventricular function, cardiac output and cavity dimensions, and should be considered in patients with **moderate to severe symptoms and a prolonged QRS** duration despite optimal medical therapy.

Adult cardiomyocytes cannot regenerate, but there is great potential to apply stem cell technology to improve cardiac function in patients with myocardial infarction and cardiomyopathy. **Skeletal myoblasts** have the capacity to perform cardiac work although they do not appear to express cardiac myocyte markers. A recent clinical study demonstrated improved left ventricular function in a patient treated with autologous myoblast implantation. Embryonic stem and bone marrow stem cells have the capacity to differentiate into cardiac myocytes. While not yet used in humans, stem cells engraft and improve cardiac function in animal models. Future studies will require delineation of function, immunogenicity and survival in humans.

The use of genetic approaches to diagnosis and treatment
The recent elucidation of the human genome and revolutions in bioinformatic analysis have demonstrated that differences in 'normal' genetic variation may have implications on disease development and therapeutics. The interaction between multiple genes (**genomics**) and the environment has a substantial impact on complex diseases such as hypertension, coronary artery disease, arrhythmias and cardiomyopathy. Single nucleotide polymorphisms (**SNPs**) in the DNA coding for subcellular structures (sarcomeres, cytoskeleton, ion channels), signalling pathways (calcineurin, protein kinases), membrane receptors (β-receptors, toll-like receptor 4), platelet glycoproteins and regulatory enzymes (renin–angiotensin, cholesterol) are associated with risk of disease. The evolving field of pharmacogenomics utilizes SNPs to understand the variability of **pharmacokinetics, therapeutic responses** and **adverse effects** of drugs.

53 Case study: heart failure

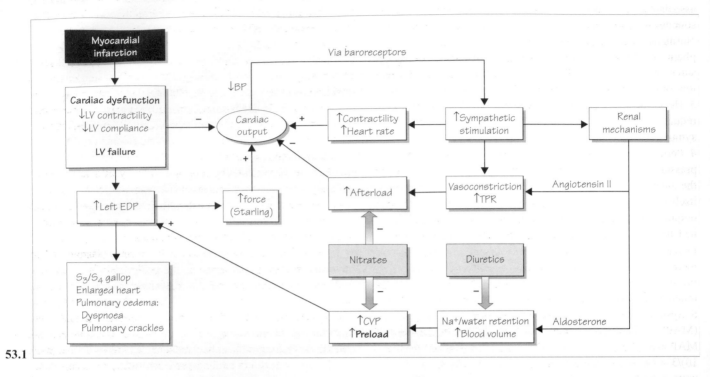

53.1

A 62-year-old man is transferred to your hospital because of recurrent chest pain and dyspnoea 5 days after suffering a large myocardial infarction. On the day of arrival he is free of chest pain but is still breathing with moderate difficulty. You obtain a chest radiograph, which confirms increased distended pulmonary vasculature, septal lines, and an enlarged heart. An echocardiogram shows an enlarged heart and an ejection fraction of 30% with minimal systolic motion of the anterior and apical portions of the heart. The patient is in normal sinus rhythm, with a heart rate of 110. Arterial blood pressure is 96/68, mean 82, respiratory rate 25/min. On cardiac auscultation you hear an S_3 gallop, an S_4 gallop, a normal S_1 and S_2, and a soft murmur that encompasses systole (holosystolic), and has uniform intensity that is heard at the apex and radiates to the left axilla. There are fine, late-inspiratory crackles (crepitations) heard about a third of the way up both lung fields. Arterial blood gases reveal a Pao_2 of 60 mmHg, $Paco_2$ of 30 mmHg, and pH of 7.37.

Questions

1 What is the left ventricular end-diastolic pressure likely to be in this patient and why?
2 What is the significance of the S_3 and S_4 gallop sounds?
3 Why is heart rate likely to be increased?
4 The arterial pressures are low. What is the peripheral vascular resistance likely to be in this case? What is the preload volume likely to be? How would similar arterial and venous loads probably affect arterial pressure in a normal heart?

5 You place a right heart catheter to assess the haemodynamics better, and find that the cardiac output is 3.0 L/min, and the right atrial pressure has a mean value of 10 mmHg. What is systemic vascular resistance? Is this normal?
6 How do abnormalities in contractile function, preload and afterload resistance play a role in this patient's current problem?
7 What might happen to cardiac output and arterial blood pressure if an arterial vasodilator was administered to this patient?
8 Would it be useful to alter contractility? In what direction? What might be a potential disadvantage of increasing contractility in this particular patient?
9 Suppose the arterial perfusion pressure during diastole could be increased while at the same time lowering it during systole. Would this intervention be useful? Why?

Answers

1 The left ventricular diastolic pressure is likely to be elevated. The recent myocardial infarction has diminished the pumping capacity of the ventricle, and to compensate the heart has filled to a larger diastolic volume to partially restore cardiac output and arterial pressures. The elevated cardiac filling pressures are reflected in the pulmonary venous pressures, and this has contributed to the pulmonary oedema. Cardiac enlargement is evident on the chest X-ray as an increase in heart size. The crackles are consistent with increased pulmonary interstitial and alveolar oedema.

2 The S_3 gallop is associated with early diastolic filling and is an indication of increased chamber stiffness. The S_4 gallop is associated with atrial contraction—late diastolic filling—and is associated with elevation of the end-diastolic pressures. Both sounds are analogous to tapping a drumhead that is pulled taut. Normally diastolic compliance is high and the chamber compliance declines if filling is increased. When end-diastolic pressures are elevated, the distensibility declines and one hears a low-pitch sound associated with filling.

3 Heart rate is likely to be increased as a compensation for reduced pump function due to the infarction. This is driven by sympathetic stimulation and vagal withdrawal.

4 Peripheral resistance is likely to be high even though arterial pressures are low. Remember that arterial pressure results from the interaction of the heart with the vascular system, and is not itself a reflection of arterial tone. In this case, reduced cardiac output would have resulted in a much lower arterial pressure had not the systemic arteries constricted. Preload volume is increased, as discussed in answer 1. If preload volume were increased and peripheral resistance increased in a normal heart, the arterial pressure would be very elevated. This can be illustrated using pressure–volume loops (see Chapter 13).

5 Systemic vascular resistance (SVR) = (mean arterial pressure (MAP) − right atrial pressure (RAP))/CO. From the data given, MAP is 82, RAP is 10, and CO is 3.0. Therefore, SVR = (82 − 10)/3 = 24. The units here are mmHg/L/min which are clinical units, but not those typically used to express resistance. The units that are more often used are dynes/s/cm^{-5}. To convert, you multiply 24 by 80 = 1920. Normal resistance is closer to 1200.

6 Net contractile function is reduced because of the recent heart injury (infarction). The heart with a heart attack is heterogeneous, with a very damaged region and remote compensating region that is closer to normal. The net effect, however, is still a decline in overall contractile function. Preload is elevated as noted, and afterload resistance increased. To improve cardiac output further and to reduce pulmonary oedema, you need to reduce preload with venodilators and diuretics, and lower afterload resistance with arterial vasodilators. Nitrates are an excellent class of drug for this purpose.

7 Cardiac output would very likely increase, and arterial pressures may not change much. If too much vasodilatation is induced, pressures will decline. However, with careful titration, one can often obtain an improvement in pump performance and coronary perfusion, and actually see a slight increase in pressure as the heart is better perfused.

8 Increasing contractile function is the last resort. One is particularly cautious in using inotropic therapy in a heart attack patient, because it is quite possible to make matters worse by increasing cardiac work and extending the territory of damage. Such patients often have coronary disease in places other than that directly responsible for the heart attack.

9 Myocardial flow occurs primarily during diastole, when myocardial pressure surrounding the arterioles is low and arterial perfusion pressure remains elevated (thanks to systemic vascular compliance and wave reflections). During systole, flow through the myocardium is inhibited by ventricular muscle contraction. So, if one had a method to enhance diastolic arterial pressures while simultaneously reducing systolic pressures, you are likely to improve cardiac perfusion while reducing ventricular load during ejection. Such a device exists and is called an **aortic counterpulsation balloon pump**. By inflating a balloon placed in the proximal descending aorta rapidly during diastole and deflating it during systole, you can augment the diastolic perfusion to the heart while improving forward output. In patients with ischaemic heart disease and reduced arterial pressures, this device is very useful indeed.

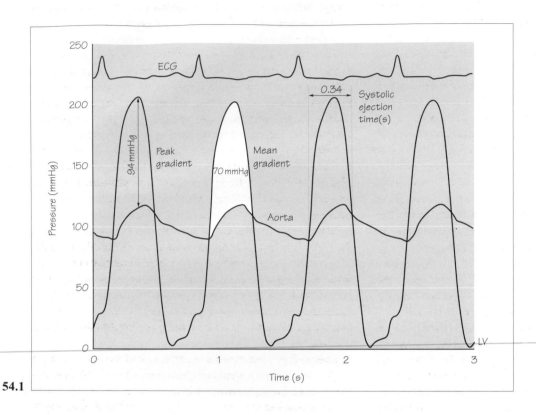

54.1

You are asked to supervise an exercise stress test on a 65-year-old man. He saw his doctor last week for exertional chest pain and mild dyspnoea. He has had chest discomfort for about a year, but the increased frequency of angina prompted him to see his doctor. He has chest pain when he walks more than one block, and if he continues he becomes breathless. He never has chest pain or dyspnoea at rest. He has no ankle swelling, orthopnoea, or paroxysmal nocturnal dyspnoea. When you examine him before the stress test, his blood pressure is 120/86, heart rate 82 and regular, jugular venous pressure 5 cmH$_2$O, and lungs are clear. His apex beat is slightly lateral to the midclavicular line and mildly sustained. He has a normal S$_1$ and a single S$_2$. An S$_4$ gallop is noted. He has a soft crescendo–decrescendo systolic murmur, best heard at the upper right sternal border, radiating to the carotids and the apex. The carotid pulses are delayed and diminished.

You call the referring doctor to discuss the signs and symptoms, cancel the stress test, and perform an echocardiogram instead.

Questions

1 What is the likely diagnosis based on the physical examination? What are the pathophysiological mechanisms underlying these findings?
2 He only had a soft systolic murmur. If you knew that his murmur last year was louder and harsher in intensity, would this

have reassured you? What could go wrong if he did do the stress test?
3 What was likely to be observed on the echocardiogram and why?

Catheterization data: The patient is formally referred to you, and you recommend valve replacement. He undergoes cardiac catheterization, and the haemodynamic data are shown in Fig. 54.1. Cardiac output is 5.2 L/min, and heart rate is 77. There is no significant coronary artery disease.

4 The aortic valve area can be estimated by the simplified formula:

Valve area = cardiac output/√pressure gradient

Based on the data given, what is his estimated valve area?
5 When admitted for surgery, he complains of chest pain. The intern orders sublingual nitroglycerin for him. Why is this a bad idea? What is the chest pain due to? What therapeutic options are available for protracted chest pain in this case?

Answers

1 He is likely to have severe aortic stenosis. The crescendo–decrescendo systolic murmur usually arises from stenosis of either the aortic or pulmonary valve. The stenotic valve creates turbulence during ejection that causes a murmur. The murmur gets louder as flow increases during ejection, then diminishes as flow decreases. This murmur is transmitted to the carotid arteries because of the high velocity of the ejected blood. The apical murmur is probably caused by high-frequency vibration of the aortic valve during ejection and can sometimes be louder than that at the sternal border.

Aortic stenosis causes left ventricular hypertrophy, which displaces the apex beat laterally. The apex beat can be sustained because the ventricle takes longer to empty. The carotid pulse contour reflects flow across the aortic valve. Because peak ejection flow is delayed and decreased in aortic stenosis, the carotid pulses are delayed and diminished.

2 The loudness of murmur depends on *flow* across the valve; therefore it may not reflect the severity of valve stenosis. In the case of aortic stenosis, other physical examination parameters are more indicative of the severity of valve stenosis. As valve area becomes smaller, the peak loudness of the murmur occurs later in systole. This is presumably due to the difficulty in opening the valve. In severe aortic stenosis left ventricular stroke volume is decreased. This manifests as low-amplitude carotid pulsation with a delayed peak (***pulsus parvus et tardus***).

Normally, the aortic valve closes before the pulmonary valve, causing splitting of S_2. During inspiration more blood volume is returned to the right heart and the pulmonary valve closes even later. The increased splitting of S_2 during inspiration is termed physiological splitting. In severe aortic stenosis, the ejection time becomes longer, and the aortic valve closes later. This may eliminate splitting of S_2 (single S_2), or create paradoxical splitting.

If this murmur was previously louder, it would suggest that flow across the valve has decreased as the stenosis worsened. Decrease in flow (lower cardiac output) is an ominous sign of a failing left ventricle or a decrease in valve size. This is not reassuring.

During exercise, blood vessels dilate and peripheral resistance decreases. When the peripheral resistance falls, the blood pressure tends to fall. Normal individuals compensate by increasing stroke volume and heart rate. However, this patient cannot increase his stroke volume because of the tight aortic valve. When blood pressure falls, coronary perfusion decreases, and the subendocardial area of the hypertrophied ventricle is not perfused adequately. As heart rate and oxygen demand increase, the supply and demand mismatch may worsen and

cause ischaemia. If a significant portion of the myocardium is affected, cardiac output can fall, causing a further drop in coronary perfusion and further worsening ischaemia. This vicious cycle can continue until the patient drops dead, an event that may not look particularly good on your record.

3 The echocardiogram showed uniform left ventricular hypertrophy. His left ventricular ejection fraction was estimated at 45%, and the aortic valve appeared calcified with impaired cusp mobility. Doppler studies showed the peak instantaneous gradient across the aortic valve was 98 mmHg with a mean gradient of 68 mmHg. Estimated aortic valve area was 0.6 cm².

The most common cause of aortic stenosis in this age group is calcific degeneration of the aortic cusps. The valvular pathology leads to left ventricular hypertrophy, a pressure gradient, and impaired emptying of the chamber, which were all demonstrated on the echocardiogram.

4 Using the formula the estimated valve area is 0.62 cm². This formula is a simplified version of the Gorlin formula, which states that the valve area is related to cardiac output, and inversely related to mean pressure gradient, systolic ejection period, and the gravitational acceleration constant. In most cases, the systolic ejection period multiplied by the acceleration constant is close to 1, so that term is not used in the estimate formula.

5 This patient's left ventricle (LV) needs all the help it can get to eject an adequate supply of blood through the pin-hole-sized aortic valve. Nitroglycerin is primarily a venodilator, and it will pool his blood in the veins. This will reduce blood returning to the heart and decrease preload. Even though the ejection fraction is only 45%, his thick LV still has high contractility and a steep end-systolic pressure–volume relation. This means that he is very sensitive to preload changes, and a slight drop in preload volume can drop blood pressure significantly, which will decrease coronary perfusion, worsen subendocardial ischaemia, decrease systolic dysfunction, lower blood pressure, and so on. Thus, nitrates are a bad idea. β-adrenergic blockers or calcium-channel blockers are also not good because they can reduce contractility. Calcium-channel blockers can also dilate peripheral arterioles and reduce blood pressure further.

What *can* you do? You may actually give some fluid to increase preload and increase cardiac output. The other mode of therapy, if the valve cannot be replaced promptly, is intra-aortic balloon counterpulsation. This can improve coronary perfusion in some cases and relieve subendocardial ischaemia.

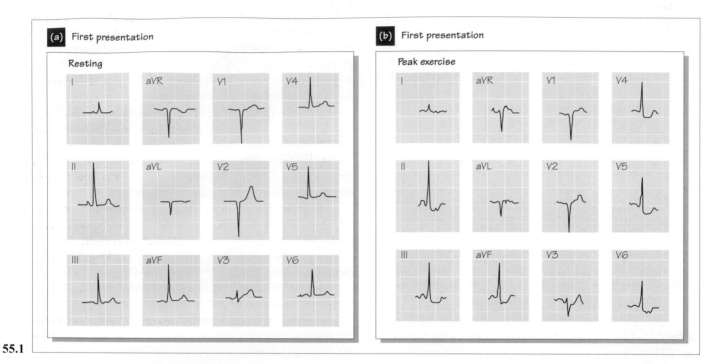

(a) First presentation

Resting

(b) First presentation

Peak exercise

55.1

A 53-year-old woman presents with a prolonged episode of chest discomfort. The discomfort is under her sternum, and is a squeezing feeling that extends to her left arm and jaws. She has had this on and off for 3 months. It usually occurs when she goes up two flights of stairs, but never when resting. Tonight, the discomfort began while walking to buy cigarettes, and lasted for 40 min. She has no known medical problems and has not seen a doctor in more than 20 years. Her last menstrual period was 4 years ago. She takes no medications. Her family history is only significant in that her father died of a heart attack when he was 74 years old.

On examination, she appears well and in no acute distress. Her height is 5 feet 6 inches (1.68 m) and weight 120 pounds (55 kg). Her blood pressure is 132/84 and heart rate 74. There is no jugular venous distension, and her lungs are clear to percussion and auscultation. Cardiac examination is normal. Her abdomen is benign, and there is no oedema. Pulses are full and equal bilaterally without thrills. An ECG shows normal sinus rhythm without abnormalities.

Questions

1 Is this angina pectoris?
2 What predisposing factors does she have for coronary artery disease (CAD)? What other risk factors might she have? Could this have been a myocardial infarction (MI)?

She is admitted for monitoring. Serial serum enzyme tests are negative, and ECG remains normal after 18 h. Fasting serum glucose is 92, and fasting lipid profile is: total cholesterol 198, HDL 36, LDL 137, and triglycerides 126. She undergoes a graded exercise test for 12 min, and has chest discomfort with the ECG abnormalities shown in Fig. 55.1(b). Her blood pressure rose from 124/78 to 180/76 at peak exercise. Her heart rate rose from 78 to 143. The chest discomfort resolved within 5 min of stopping exercise, and the ECG returned to normal. Coronary angiography showed a focal 70% narrowing in the right coronary artery and a focal 30% narrowing in the left anterior descending artery (LAD). She is treated with anti-ischaemic medicines, advised on low-cholesterol diets and aerobic exercise, instructed on the use of sublingual nitroglycerin, started on aspirin and atenolol, and discharged. She agrees to stop smoking. She will return for follow-up in 7 days for another exercise test.

3 What serum enzymes are useful in diagnosing myocardial damage?
4 Why not perform angioplasty on the coronary lesions?
5 Her cholesterol is not high. Why a low-cholesterol diet? Would lowering blood cholesterol help her existing CAD? What other risk factors can she modify?
6 Why perform a follow-up exercise test?

Second presentation: The patient does well on the medicines and stops smoking. She has no chest discomfort even during vigorous exercise. However, within th   s awakened from sleep by the same ches   lycerin is

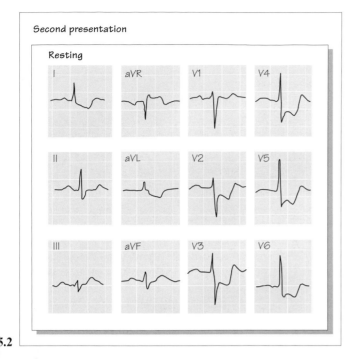

Second presentation

Resting

I	aVR	V1	V4
II	aVL	V2	V5
III	aVF	V3	V6

5.2

ineffective, she is brought to hospital. Her ECG is shown in Fig. 55.2. She is given oxygen, aspirin, intravenous nitroglycerin and heparin, and her chest discomfort then recedes. It lasted for 35 min. Because of recurrent chest discomfort in hospital, she has another coronary angiogram. This shows the same 70% narrowing in the right coronary artery, but the 30% LAD narrowing has now grown to 99%. Cardiac enzymes are still negative.

7 What does the new ECG show? What is your diagnosis? How is the pathophysiology of the current chest discomfort different from her previous effort-related angina?

8 Do the ECG abnormalities correlate with the coronary angiogram? What is the 'culprit' lesion? How could the LAD lesion progress so fast? Why use aspirin and heparin? How about thrombolytic agents?

Answers

1 This sounds like angina. The location, radiation and type of discomfort are consistent with cardiac ischaemic pain.

2 Her risk factors for CAD are smoking and being postmenopausal. Her family history is *not* positive for premature CAD, because her father was 74 when he had his MI. She does not have hypertension. We do not yet know her cholesterol levels, or whether she is diabetic.

The traditional dividing line between 'angina' and possible MI is 30 min of discomfort. Because her discomfort lasted more than 30 min, it is possible she suffered an MI, even with

a normal ECG. To determine whether a MI occurred, look for evidence of myocardial damage such as cardiac-specific serum enzymes.

3 The most commonly used enzyme is creatine kinase. A rise in serum levels of the cardiac specific (MB) isoform is seen with myocardial damage. Cardiac troponins are useful in confirming myocardial damage.

4 She does not have unstable angina at this point, and her effort tolerance is reasonable. Such patients have a good prognosis whether they take medicines or have single-vessel angioplasty. A recent study showed that angioplasty was no better than medicines for single-vessel CAD.

5 Her cholesterol was not high, but recent studies indicate that lowering LDL cholesterol below ~110 mg/dl may stabilize coronary lesions and possibly cause regression of CAD. However, greater effects were seen on reduced incidence of unstable angina or MI. These may be due to reducing the lipid-rich area of plaques and making them less susceptible to rupture.

The most important thing was to stop smoking. Reducing cholesterol is a secondary prevention. Another risk factor is lack of oestrogen. Postmenopausal women with CAD may benefit from hormone replacement therapy.

6 Reasons for exercise testing are: diagnosis; prognosis; and to test effectiveness of treatment. Here, we want to know if her anti-anginal regimen is adequate.

7 The ECG shows marked ST segment depression in the precordial (V1–V6) and lateral (I and aVL) leads. She has cardiac ischaemia, due either to unstable angina or a MI. The chest discomfort occurred during sleep, so it is unstable angina. She could additionally have an MI, as ST segment elevation is not always present in MI.

Cardiac ischaemia occurs when myocardial oxygen demand exceeds supply. This typically happens with exertion in CAD patients, because bloodflow through the stenosis is usually adequate during rest. Rest ischaemia is caused when the oxygen supply falls below that required for even basal myocardial metabolic needs. This implies a more occlusive lesion, such as unstable angina. It is believed that unstable angina is initiated by plaque rupture, causing aggregation of platelets and fibrin deposition. This can cause not only stenosis, but also vasospasm.

8 The angiogram suggests the 'culprit' is the LAD lesion. It is tighter, and stenotic enough to cause rest angina. The ECG abnormalities are consistent with the ischaemic area being that served by the LAD. Unstable angina involves platelets and the clotting cascade. Thus it makes sense to use inhibitors of platelet aggregation (aspirin) and anticoagulants (heparin). Clot formation and dissolution are dynamic processes, and although aspirin and heparin cannot directly disperse clots, they can promote resolution. Thrombolytics make theoretical sense, but in trials no improvement in outcome of unstable angina patients was seen, and morbidity was *higher*.

56 Case studies: arrhythmias

Case 1

Initial presentation: A 64-year-old man with a history of long-standing hypertension and diabetes presents complaining of shortness of breath and weakness. He has orthopnoea but no chest pain. His physical examination is notable for a heart rate of 150 beats/min, a blood pressure of 100/70, and a respiratory rate of 24. There are bilateral crackles a third of the way up the lung fields, the first heart sound is soft, and there is a summation gallop. His ECG is shown in Fig. 56.1(a). Carotid sinus massage then changes the rhythm to the one shown in Fig. 56.1(b).

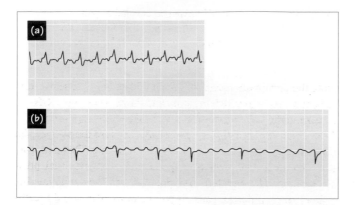

Figure 56.1 (a) Lead II. Atrial flutter with 2 : 1 conduction. Heart rate 150 beats/min. (b) Lead II. Arial flutter after carotid sinus massage. Note the characteristic sawtooth pattern of flutter waves, and AV conduction of 4 : 1 to 6 : 1.

Questions

1 What is the ventricular rate in Fig. 56.1(a)? Is this a ventricular or supraventricular arrhythmia?
2 Based on the effect of carotid sinus massage, what is the diagnosis? How does carotid sinus massage affect the ventricular response?
3 What pharmacological agents can be used to slow the ventricular response?

Results of treatment: The patient is admitted to hospital and begun on digitalis and amiodarone. The next morning he feels better, but his pulse is irregularly irregular with an apical pulse of 110 and a radial pulse of 70. An ECG is shown in Fig. 56.2.

4 What is the rhythm now? Is the change from the day before common?
5 Is the current antiarrhythmic regimen appropriate?
6 What other therapy may be indicated? Why?

Answers

1 The ventricular rate is 150 beats/min. The narrow QRS complex implies that the tachycardia involves the atrioventricular

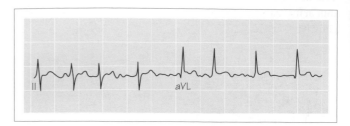

Figure 56.2 Leads II and aVL. Atrial flutter has degenerated into atrial fibrillation. Note the irregularity of the ventricular rate, indicated by the varying intervals between the QRS complexes.

node (AVN), and is therefore supraventricular. The differential diagnosis for this tachycardia includes AV nodal re-entrant tachycardia, atrial flutter, or sinus tachycardia. Atrial fibrillation is unlikely because the rhythm is regular.
2 Carotid sinus massage demonstrates the sawtooth pattern of flutter waves, particularly in the inferior leads (II, III, aVF). This proves that the initial rhythm was atrial flutter with 2 : 1 conduction (i.e. only one of every two atrial waves is conducted through the AVN to the ventricle). Because the flutter waves have a rate of nearly 300 beats/min, the ventricular rate is 150 beats/min. Carotid sinus massage increases vagal tone, slowing conduction through the AVN and increasing AV block.
3 β-blockers, digoxin, Ca^{2+}-channel blockers and adenosine slow conduction through the AVN. This slows the ventricular rate, allowing adequate time for left ventricular filling, and relieving the symptoms of left heart failure (shortness of breath, weakness, orthopnoea).
4 This is atrial fibrillation; note the irregularly irregular ventricular rate. Atrial flutter is an unstable rhythm, and commonly degenerates into atrial fibrillation.
5 Yes. Amiodarone and digoxin are commonly used to treat atrial arrhythmias. Digoxin helps to slow the ventricular rate by increasing vagal tone at the AVN. Amiodarone similarly helps to slow the ventricular response. Amiodarone is also used to cardiovert patients with atrial arrhythmias back into sinus rhythm and/or help maintain sinus rhythm once they have been electrically cardioverted.
6 Patients with intermittent or persistent atrial fibrillation should receive anticoagulation because of the risk of embolic stroke. In this patient, who seems to be having his first episode of atrial fibrillation, electrical cardioversion should be attempted if amiodarone does not convert the rhythm to sinus.

Case 2

Initial presentation: A 55-year-old man presents with a 24-h history of shortness of breath and palpitations. He has mild dizziness and diaphoresis. There is no prior record of MI, but he has longstanding hypertension and cigarette smoking. His blood pressure is 80/52, heart rate is 186 beats/min and regular, and his respiratory rate is 26. There are crackles bilaterally, jugular venous pressure (JVP) is raised, and a III/VI holosystolic murmur at the apex radiates to the axilla but not the neck. His ECG is shown in Fig. 56.3.

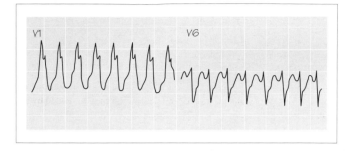

Figure 56.3 Leads V1 and V6. Ventricular tachycardia. Heart rate 186 beats/min. The QRS complex is abnormally wide. There is a large primary R wave in lead V1, and exaggerated R wave, leading to an R/S ratio < 1, in V6.

Questions

1 What does the III/VI holosystolic murmur indicate?
2 Is this tachycardia more likely supraventricular or ventricular? Why? What is the axis and the QRS morphology?
3 Why is he short of breath and hypotensive? Why is his JVP elevated?
4 What would be appropriate treatment?

Results of treatment: The patient receives lidocaine. This fails to convert him to sinus rhythm and he is therefore electrically cardioverted. The resulting ECG is shown in Fig. 56.4.

5 What is the rhythm now?
6 What is the likely cause of his acute presentation?
7 What would be the appropriate evaluation with this information?

Answers

1 This indicates a moderate murmur of mitral regurgitation (see Chapter 50).
2 This rhythm is most likely ventricular in origin. When a patient has a wide-complex tachycardia, the differential diagnosis is ventricular tachycardia (VT) vs supraventricular tachycardia with aberrant conduction (i.e. the tachycardia is conducted with a bundle branch block). A wide variety of clinical and ECG criteria aid in distinguishing between these possibilities. The most important clinical criterion is whether the patient has a history of heart disease (see below). If this is the case, and in particular if there is a history of MI, the most likely origin of the tachycardia is ventricular, because an infarct creates a substrate for re-entry. ECG criteria which suggest a ventricular origin include: (i) a very wide QRS complex; (ii) an extreme axis; (iii) evidence of atrial-ventricular dissociation; (iv) certain specific QRS morphologies. This patient's QRS morphology is that of a right bundle.

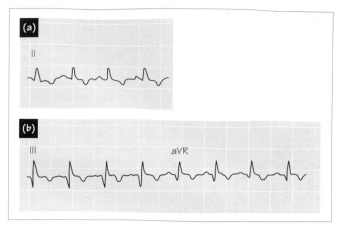

Figure 56.4 Leads II, III, aVR. After cardioversion, patient restored to sinus rhythm. Heart rate 95 beats/min. Note the exaggerated Q waves and elevation of the ST segment, indicating an old inferior wall MI.

Note the terminal S waves in V6, and the R in V1. The extreme axis, the very wide QRS duration and the morphology (R/S < 1 in V6 and the large primary R in V1) suggest the rhythm is VT.
3 He is short of breath and hypotensive because the tachycardia does not allow enough time for ventricular filling. Therefore cardiac output is low, causing hypotension, and left atrial pressure is high. The high left atrial pressure has backed up into his pulmonary capillaries, causing pulmonary oedema and breathlessness. His increased JVP is caused by raised central venous pressure, indicative of inadequate right ventricular function. His arrhythmia is therefore causing congestive heart failure.
4 Treatment requires cardioversion to sinus rhythm with either appropriate drugs (lidocaine, procainamide, or amiodarone) or electrical cardioversion. Because this patient's symptoms indicate that his arrhythmia is causing his heart to fail, immediate conversion to sinus rhythm is mandatory. Therefore in this case electrical cardioversion is preferable.
5 The rhythm is now sinus, with the rate of 95 beats/min.
6 He has evidence on his ECG of an inferior wall MI (note the Q waves in leads II, III, aVF with slight ST elevation). The aetiology of his ventricular tachycardia is likely to be re-entry into left ventricular (LV) scar caused by an undetected recent acute MI.
7 Following stabilization, appropriate treatment includes evaluation of LV function and of coronary anatomy.

In this case, the patient had severe inoperable coronary artery disease and poor LV function. Because a poor ejection fraction identifies high risk for recurrent VT and sudden death, the patient underwent electrophysiology testing and was readily inducible into hypotensive VT. This indicated: (i) that he was at a high risk of spontaneously developing VT again; (ii) that his tachycardia was fast enough to lower his cardiac output dangerously. His already poor LV function meant that he would not be able to tolerate tachycardia. He therefore subsequently underwent successful placement of an internal cardioverter-defibrillator and has since been stable.

Index